WILD TEA

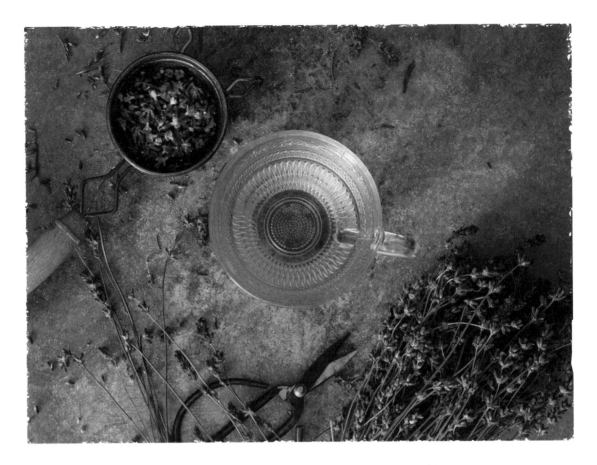

This edition published in 2020 by Stackpole Books
An imprint of The Rowman & Littlefield Publishing Group, Inc.
4501 Forbes Blvd., Ste. 200
Lanham, MD 20706
www.stackpolebooks.com

Distributed by NATIONAL BOOK NETWORK
800-462-6420

British Library Cataloguing in Publication Information available

Library of Congress Cataloging-in-Publication Data available

Library of Congress Control Number: 2019957451
ISBN 978-0-8117-3894-1 (cloth : alk. paper)

The paper used in this publication meets the minimum requirements of
American National Standard for Information Sciences—Permanence of
Paper for Printed Library Materials, ANSI/NISO Z39.48-1992.

First Edition

DISCLAIMER

Although every effort has been made to make
the information in this book as correct and as
clear as possible, the author and publisher do not
assume and hereby disclaim any liability to any
party for any damage, injury, illness, or loss of
life caused as a result of mistakes in the text or
images within this book (or mistakes by anyone
translating or interpreting the text or images).
This book is meant as only a general beverage
guide and is neither a plant identification guide
or a substitute for professional medical advice.
Any information given should be read with the
discretion of the reader.

All images © Richard Hood and Nick Moyle
2020, except: © Eddison Books Ltd 2020: pages
2, 4–5, 22–23, 24, 29, 49, 53, 56, 59, 61, 62, 71,
75, 77, 81, 85, 87, 89, 91, 97, 99, 101, 103, 104,
120tl, 120bl, 120br, 121, 122, 124, 125, 126, 127,
129, 131, 132, 134, 139, 140, 143, 145, 146, 147, 148,
152, 155, 157, 161, 163, 168 / Shutterstock: page 7
ArtSyslik, 38 Sunvik, 165 mama_mia.

WILD TEA

GROW, GATHER, BREW & BLEND
40 INGREDIENTS & 30 RECIPES FOR
HEALTHFUL HERBAL TEAS

NICK MOYLE AND RICHARD HOOD

STACKPOLE
BOOKS
Guilford, Connecticut

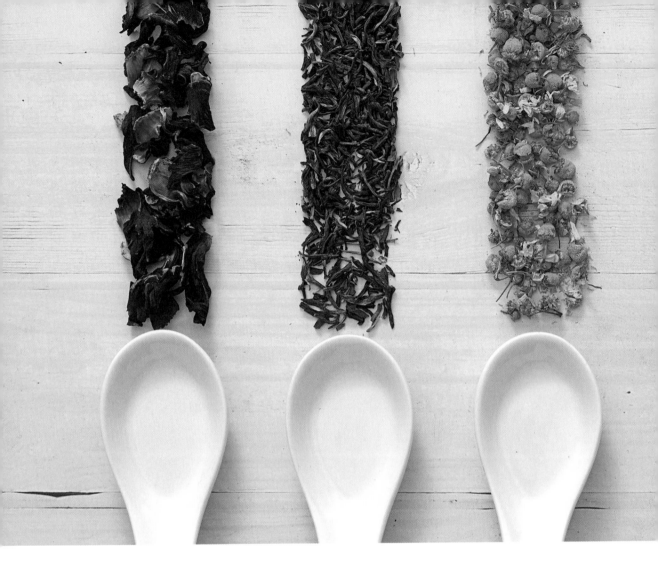

Contents

26 Top 40 Ingredients

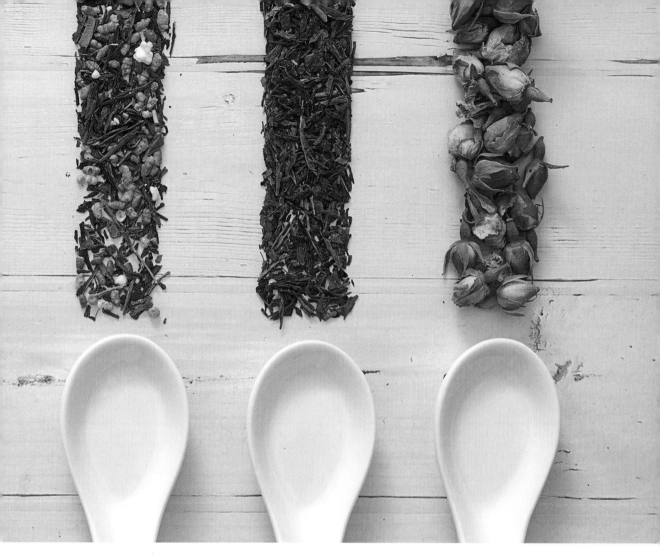

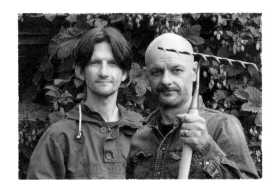

Foreword

Hi there, we are Nick and Rich, also known as the Two Thirsty Gardeners, and we grow and forage for things to turn into beverages. Our first book, *Brew it Yourself*, featured boozy beverages, so we thought it was time to sober up with teas for our second book. We live in Somerset, England, where the countryside is well stocked with forage-worthy ingredients, and we also grow whatever our lazy gardening methods allow—Nick in his yard and Rich in his community garden.

So pull up a comfortable chair, pour yourself a cup of tea, sit down, and relax as we tell you all about wild tea. You could, of course, jump to the recipes and launch straight into brewing a cup of tea, but there are a few things you might want to know before you do. Are you sitting comfortably? Then let us begin ...

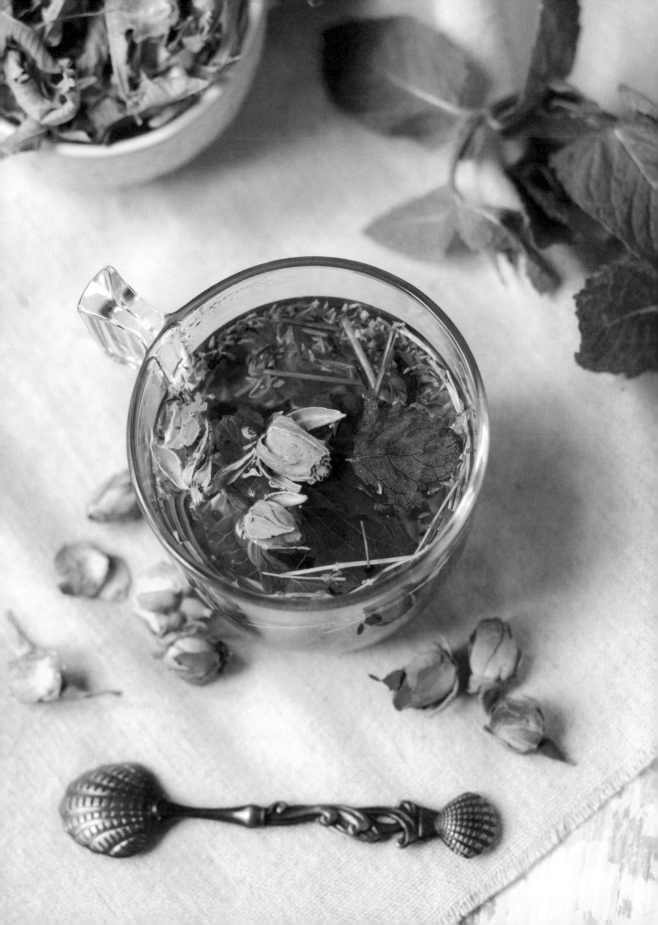

What Is Wild Tea?

We use the term "wild tea" to cover infusions and decoctions (see below) made from ingredients other than "true" teas that come from the *Camellia sinensis* plant (see *page 20*). These flowers, leaves, seeds, fruits, and roots can be turned into a huge range of delicious drinks, usually with the same minimal effort as brewing a regular cup of tea, giving you an infinite range of flavors to fill your teapots, cups, and mugs.

A number of the ingredients featured in this book can be found in the wild, and many more can be cultivated in the wilds of your own yard (or even a flowerpot or window box for those who have limited space). For us, their "wildness" is just as much about the experimental process of deviating from familiar teas and into new taste territories.

To get you going, we've picked out our forty favorite wild tea ingredients, chosen not only for their great taste, but also because they're easy to grow or forage, or they are so essential we couldn't leave them out. We've also highlighted more ingredients in the Best of the Rest section, focusing on those that didn't quite make our top forty, along with some other interesting and unusual plants with a teatime tale to tell.

For those of you who want some inspiration for blending teas, we have a whole section on just that. We've also got some extra-special tea and coffee recipes that require a little more effort than simply infusing—these include sun teas, iced teas, bubble teas, and other brewing delights.

However, before all of that, we want to give you a few pointers on how to grow, forage, and dry your own ingredients, and explain some of the key tea terminology so you'll be an expert in no time. Now, isn't it time for another cup of tea?

TEAS, TISANES, INFUSIONS, AND DECOCTIONS

A good cup of tea comes in many guises. The term "wild tea" encompasses all of the following tea-type drinks:

Teas: There has been some debate about whether herbal, fruit, and botanical teas should technically be labeled as "tea." The word "tea" comes from the common name given to *Camellia sinensis*—the "tea plant"—so people will argue that it shouldn't be applied to beverages that are made from other ingredients. However, we think language is flexible enough to let us ignore this technicality and refer to all of our infusions and decoctions as "tea."

Tisanes: The French already have a word for these drinks—*tisane.** Although it's occasionally used in English, it sounds too fancy for common folk like us to use with any confidence, so we're sticking with tea.

Infusions: In tea terms, this is the name for a drink made by pouring boiling water over your chosen ingredients and then letting them steep to extract their flavors.

Decoctions: This term is used to describe drinks that have been made by simmering ingredients in boiling water. This method is used to extract flavor from items that are more reluctant to give up their goodness by infusion alone.

COFFEE AND MILK

We also have a few recipes that tell you how to make coffee and milk substitutes. Although no coffee beans or cows were involved in the making of these drinks, we will refer to them as "coffee" and "milk," because coming up with alternative names is just too confusing.

STORE-BOUGHT INGREDIENTS

We find that growing or foraging for your own ingredients is part of the fun of wild tea making. But you don't have to rely on such wild ways to source the goods—rummaging around in stores is a perfectly acceptable method for gathering your tea-making bounties. Even among our forty favorite ingredients, there are a few entries that we neither grow or forage for ourselves (lemon being a notable example), but we deem them too important and tasty to ignore.

You'll be able to make a large number of these teas from ingredients found in a large grocery store, and just about every other item will be available online (particularly in dried form), so you can infuse and decoct without even leaving the house, let alone getting your fingers muddy.

If you're lucky enough to have access to a good herbalist or apothecary, these are the ideal places to source dried ingredients. You can see and sniff (and maybe even have a nibble) before you buy and can usually get whatever amount you want measured out, allowing for you to experiment with the flavors before stocking up on larger quantities.

HEALTH AND WELL-BEING

Although many of the ingredients in this book have well-known health and well-being benefits, we're not medical experts and tend to take some of the more remarkable claims with a large dose of skepticism. Even if, for example, you believe that black currant leaves can cure aching joints, you would probably need to take the teas as regular doses over a period of time (just like prescription medicines), in which

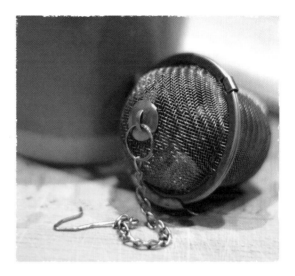

case we advise first talking with your physician. It is also the case that not all vitamins are water soluble, so simply dunking an ingredient in hot water won't necessarily release all of its good stuff.

We've highlighted some medical claims surrounding each of our main ingredients to help to build a bigger picture about the reasons for their popularity, but mostly we've included ingredients for their flavor, not their health benefits.

Disclaimer: It's worth mentioning that, as with consuming anything, some of the ingredients featured may cause unwanted side effects, particularly if you ingest a lot of them or start to use them regularly. Anyone with an existing medical condition, or who is pregnant or breastfeeding, should be particularly cautious. Some people can have an allergy to certain ingredients, so treat everything with caution. It's also worth noting that, with many of our ingredients, there are multiple varieties of the same species, so be especially careful to check that the one you're using is safe to consume. If you're not absolutely sure, always err on the side of cautious.

---

* *Just as you could argue that "tea" should only refer to drinks made from the tea plant, you could say that "tisane" should only refer to drinks made from barley, because the word derives from the Greek* ptisane, *meaning "peeled barley." We told you language was flexible.*

Brewing Basics

Making tea is not exactly rocket science, but here are some Two Thirsty Gardener tips to make sure you get the best from your ingredients.

HOW MUCH?

The quantities given in this book are only guidelines. You may like your tea stronger, lighter, sweeter, or served in another way. Think about the many different ways people drink black tea and coffee, and then apply these same variations to wild teas. It can take several cups until you hit on your own personal preferences.

DRIED OR FRESH?

Where possible, we have indicated whether ingredients should be dried or used fresh. These are our preferences, but in the spirit of this book, we urge you to experiment. For example, we like the savory edge that dried rose petals can bring, but you may prefer the floral sweetness of freshly picked specimens for your own herbal brews.

RELEASE THE FLAVOR

When using fresh ingredients, some plants require some encouragement to release their essential oils and flavors. To do this, rub them briefly between the palms of your hands before dropping them into your teapot or cup.

WHAT TEMPERATURE?

Completely oxidized teas, such as black tea, require freshly boiled water poured at 212°F to fully release their flavor. However, for a first-rate brew made from more delicate ingredients, such as green teas (and most of the ingredients in this book), let your water cool for a few minutes before pouring.

TEATIME(ING)

As a general rule, steep your concoctions for five minutes before tasting. If you feel your brew needs a little more flavor, give it another five minutes and have another sip.

TEA-MAKING KIT

We've listed below the key items you'll need to aid you in your tea-making experiments:

INFUSERS

These devices will hold your tea ingredients in situ while they infuse, letting the flavors flow but stopping particles from floating around in your chosen vessel. They come in various guises, from elaborate infuser wands to reusable silicone tea bags. Our tool of choice is the no-nonsense "tea globe," a stainless steel mesh ball attached to a chain for easy removal.

If you plan to prepare and serve your herbal brews on a larger scale, teapots with built-in infusers are worth a look. You can also buy an infuser thermos for brewing on the go. Steeping and brewing times will be haphazard, but for making simple mint teas in your community garden, they are just the ticket.

STRAINERS

If you choose not to follow the infuser route, it's always good practice to strain your brews before serving. Small, cup-size ones that rest on the rim are best, but a fine-mesh strainer used for baking can be an effective, albeit less graceful, alternative.

STRAWS

For elegant sampling of iced teas and cold-served beverages, straws are ideal. Stainless steel ones are best for the environment, and you'll need to source some wide-bored ones if you want to try our Bubble Tea (see *page 162*).

CUTTING BOARD

A concave hardwood board will help you prep without spilling your precious ingredients. Combine it with a semicircle herb chopper to rock and roll through ingredients with precision and speed.

MORTAR AND PESTLE

You'll need one of these to help grind up some of the more resilient ingredients. Don't forget to rest the mortar (the cup part) on a cutting board or tea towel when grinding to prevent damage to your kitchen surfaces.

MEASURING EQUIPMENT

The measurements in this book are only for guidance, so you don't need to get too hung up on precision, but a set of stainless steel measuring spoons and measuring cups will be a handy kitchen ally. Start with the measurements given in the recipes, and then adjust them to suit your tastes—you may want to use more or less of certain ingredients, so feel free to experiment with the quantities.

SLOTTED SPOON

It is essential for high-speed stirring and for the removal of unwanted objects that would otherwise ruin your cup of tea.

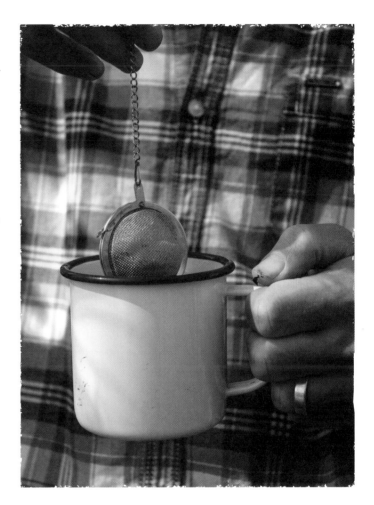

STERILIZATION

When making and storing the syrups in this book, sterilize your chosen vessels carefully before use to prevent unwanted cultures from forming and spoiling your syrup. Put cleaned and rinsed jars or bottles, right side up, into a stockpot or boiling-water canner with a rack on the bottom, along with the lids (but not screw bands if using jars with two-part lids). Add enough water so there is an inch about the vessels, bring the water to a boil, and boil for 10 minutes plus an extra minute for every 1,000 feet of elevation, then reduce the heat and keep them in the water until needed.

Drying Ingredients

While some ingredients taste best fresh, many more are just as good—if not better—when dried. If you want to create blends and store teas long after their harvest season has ended, then drying them first is essential.

HOW TO DRY YOUR INGREDIENTS

There are many reasons why you might want to dry your wild tea ingredients. Besides enabling you to store them for longer, they will be easier to crumble or grind into smaller pieces, making them more suitable for infusers and homemade tea bags. Dried ingredients provide maximum blending opportunities (which is particularly useful when combining ingredients from different seasons) and, in many instances, drying intensifies flavor for a better tasting brew.

There are two main things that ingredients need to dry successfully: heat and air. Heat extracts the water, but air circulating around the ingredients throughout the process will dry them more evenly and disperse any moisture, preventing it from building up where it's not wanted.

Successful drying can be achieved naturally by placing your ingredients somewhere warm in the open (for example, a sunroom, greenhouse, or even a hot windowsill), or by using a heat source, such as an oven or a specialized dehydrator. Delicate ingredients (small flowers and thin leaves) dry quickly, so the open air method is often best, and thicker leaves, fruits, and roots will generally benefit from the more consistently hot temperatures provided by ovens or dehydrators. Some leaves and flowers can be dried while still on their stems, enabling you to tie them together and suspend them, then pluck the goods off when finished.

To let air circulate freely, dehydrators are fitted with specially designed trays so you can leave your ingredients unattended throughout the drying process. Oven users will have to lay their ingredients out on a baking sheet and regularly turn them to make sure they dry evenly.

To create the most flavorsome dried teas, it's best to start the process as soon as possible after picking. Always wash ingredients first and remove as much water as possible by patting with a clean dish towel or paper towels. Try to dry ingredients of a similar size and thickness to make sure everything is ready at the same time and, for larger items, slice them thinly so they will dry more evenly and in a shorter amount of time.

Items are completely dried and ready for storage when there's no moisture left in them—leaves and flowers will lose their flexibility and crumble easily, while thicker items will become firm and dry and can be easily ground. The best place to store your newly dried tea-making ingredients is in a well-sealed opaque can, jar, or bag in a cool, dark place.

DRYING CITRUS FRUITS

When drying citrus fruits, you can choose to slice the whole fruit into disks (often referred to as wheels) or just peel off and use the outer rind. The former will provide you with impressive looking disks containing all the flavors of the fruit, but they will include the bitterness of the pith, which can tarnish some delicate tea blends.

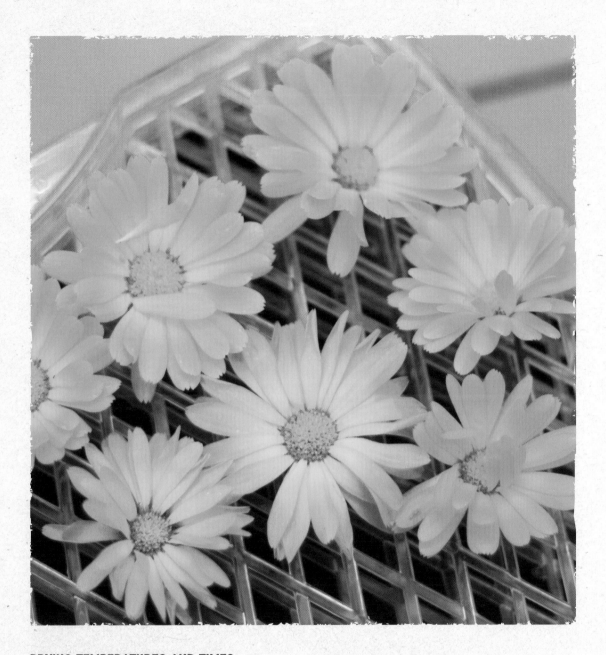

DRYING TEMPERATURES AND TIMES

We haven't included drying temperatures or times in this book, because there are too many variables to give consistent results. These factors can include obvious things, such as the size and thickness of your ingredients, or the amount of moisture in each item and even the humidity levels in the air.

As a guide to temperatures, a range of 105–165°F will cover most ingredients in a slow, steady manner. The lower end is good for delicate leaves and flowers, the upper end for juicy fruits and roots. The trick is to regularly check your ingredients while they're drying so you capture them at their peak.

What to Grow

Growing your own ingredients can be an incredibly rewarding activity and, no matter where you live in the world, you'll have a decent range of plants to choose from. You don't need a green thumb to be successful, but for those who are new to gardening, here are a few words of advice to get you up and running.

GETTING STARTED

When deciding what to grow, it's worth taking into consideration the natural habitat of each plant and choosing things that thrive in similar conditions to your garden. You can, of course, push the boundaries and introduce plants from other regions, but try to replicate their natural conditions as much as possible. For example, Mediterranean plants will probably want sunshine and good drainage; tropical plants will benefit from warmth all year round; and woodland plants will thrive better in the damp, shady recesses of your yard.

Some folk go to great lengths to grow their favorite fruits, vegetables, and flowers, but we prefer to adopt a much lazier attitude toward gardening: trial and error. If something refuses to grow without our full attention, then we move on and give the space to something else instead. After all, we want time to enjoy relaxing in our yard instead of spending all our time weeding, pruning, fertilizing, and nurturing.

Within this book, you'll find a huge range of plants that will suit any style of yard, be it a rambling wildlife haven, a formal outdoor space, or a collection of flowerpots perched on a balcony. There's always room for a few tea-giving plants, whether they are trees, flowers, vegetables, or herbs—and we've covered them all.

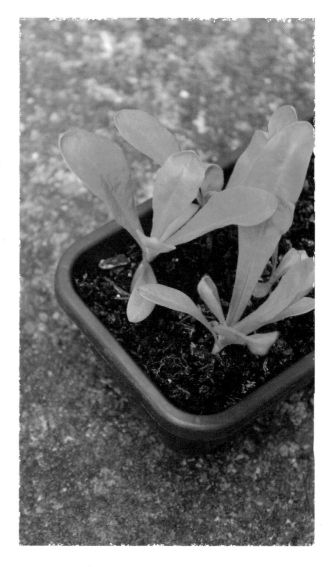

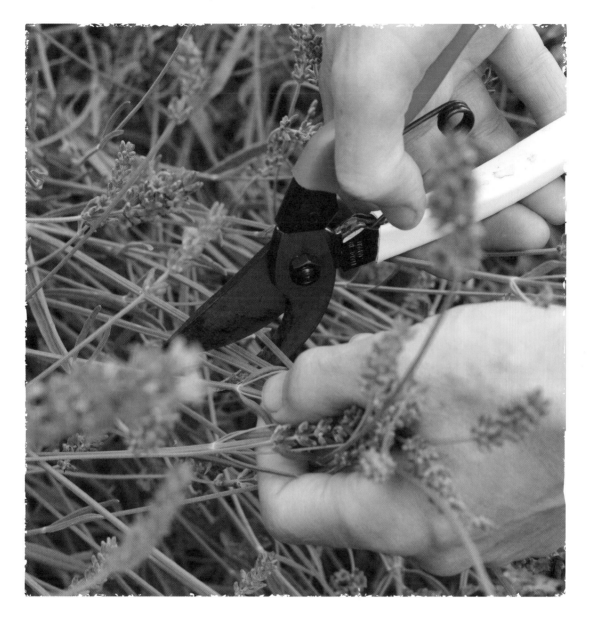

There are three main ways to get new plants into your yard: sowing seed, propagating them from an existing plant, or buying an established plant.

SOWING SEED

This is an inexpensive way of adding a lot of plants to your yard, and the range of seeds at your local garden center or nursery is almost certainly going to be bigger than their range of established plants.

Not everything grows well from seed, and it can take more time and effort than other methods, but watching a tiny seedling turn into a big, leafy crop is extremely rewarding. Sowing seed is most valuable for annuals, plants that are sown, grow, flower, fruit, and die all within one year.

For seed-sowing beginners, we recommend flowers, such as marigold and chamomile, or some vegetables, with beet being a good option to start with.

You can spend a long time searching the Internet and reading books on how to best grow your chosen seeds but, more often than not, the concise advice printed on the back of the seed packet is the best.

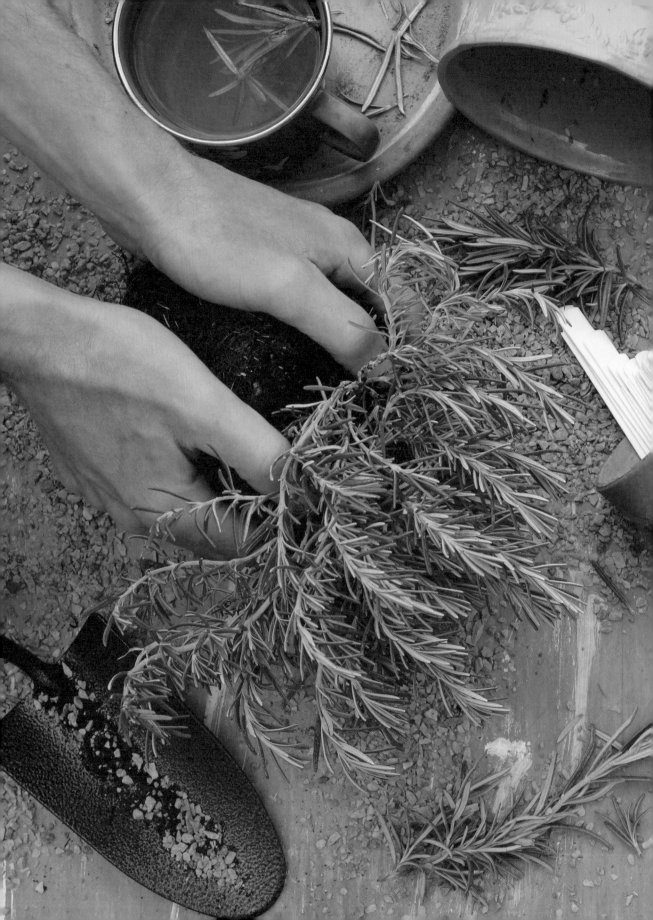

TAKING CUTTINGS OR DIVIDING PLANTS

If you want to multiply some of your favorite plants, taking cuttings or dividing them is a free way to achieve this. The methods won't work for everything, so do some research to find out if "propagation" is achievable for what you want to grow. A cutting is simply a snippet of plant growth that is allowed to develop new roots, either by planting it in a potting mix or first putting it into water. Some herbs, including mint, lavender, and rosemary, are easy to cultivate by this method, and fruit bushes, such as black currants, can also be grown in this way.

Dividing involves breaking up an established plant into smaller pieces. It is suitable for some plants that spread out their root system as they grow and don't mind being dug up and chopped. Bee balm, mint, lemongrass, and rhubarb can all be divided easily.

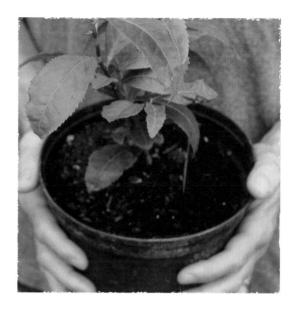

BUYING ESTABLISHED PLANTS

Of course, the easiest method to quickly fill a patch of yard or a container is to buy an established plant. It will be more expensive than the other methods but will provide you with instant results for minimum effort. If you're not too sure on how or when to plant your new purchases, make sure you buy them from a reputable garden center or nursery and ask the staff for advice. You should also check that your plant looks healthy, with no yellowing of the leaves, and that it hasn't become pot-bound—a condition where the roots grow too large for the container and wrap around the inside of the flowerpot. Plants that are in a poor condition in their containers are less likely to thrive when they are planted into the ground.

WHAT WE GROW

Nick grows a lot of his tea-making plants in flowerpots—mint, lemon verbena, and bay all sit next to his kitchen door for quick access to a fresh cup. He also stuffs his flower borders with other wild tea ingredients, including lavender, hyssop, marigold, chamomile, and fennel. Even some wild plants, notably yarrow and a self-seeded elderflower, have been allowed space in the yard. He also has a small greenhouse, which is ideal for sowing seed early in the year and has room for a few fruit bushes and some wild strawberries, while a rampant sage plant threatens to smother it all.

Rich is the proud keeper of a plot at a community garden, which is home to his five prized apple trees, a tangled mass of raspberry canes, and most of his wild tea ingredients. He grows produce in raised beds and one is entirely for tea ingredients, including chamomile, borage, and marigold (some of which came from Nick's greenhouse). Having the extra space at a community garden also gives him the opportunity to experiment with some of the more unusual ingredients in this book. He has given one bed to three brewing grains: barley, oats, and wheat. Around the edges of his plot, Rich has carefully nurtured and protected several wild plants, including nettles, dandelions, and a rambling rose.*

* *Some folk might consider these invasive weeds. Not us.*

Rules of Foraging

You can grow many of the ingredients mentioned in this book in your yard but, for some, you'll need to venture out beyond the gate and do some foraging. Plant finding and identification is a skill that takes patience and a sharp eye, but a few days out and about in the wilderness with a decent plant identification book or phone app can provide some guidance. Better yet, join a local nature group or enroll in a foraging class run by people in the know. Before long, you'll start to see the countryside as a giant tea caddy and be able to see a berry-bearing elder from many yards away.

THE FIVE GOLDEN RULES OF FORAGING

Before heading out with goodie bag in hand, there are a few essential rules that the aspiring forager must adhere to for safe and responsible foraging:

1. Mind Where You Pick

The laws governing foraging are different around the world, with gray areas aplenty. In the United States, laws vary state by state. Wandering over private property without permission is, of course, trespass and you should steer well clear of nature reserves, conservation areas, and areas of scientific interest. Use common sense when foraging and, wherever possible, first seek permission.

2. Mind What You Are Picking

Some plants are lethal to ingest, and there are countless horror stories of foraging folk undergoing hospital treatment after gobbling a wrongly identified plant. You may also unwittingly pull up a protected plant species, so be 100 percent sure of your quarry.

3. Pick in Moderation

Don't descend on and decimate a plant like a plague of locusts. Leave plenty behind for the birds, insects, and mammals to enjoy. It is, after all, their pantry that you are raiding.

4. Wash Before Use

Insects, insecticides, and pollution are not conducive to a nice cup of tea. Makes sure you always rid your plants of any contamination—visible or otherwise—before using it. Discard anything that looks rotten or has an undesirable smell.

5. Avoid Low-Level Picking on Walkways

Plants that live beside public thoroughfares will be at the mercy of every passing pooch. Always forage higher than a dog can cock its leg.

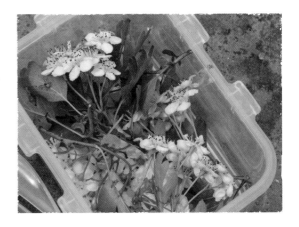

FORAGING KIT CHECKLIST

Now that you know the golden rules of foraging, you need to make sure you have the right equipment with you, so you can collect and store your bounty in the best way:

☑ *Containers and Bags*

You'll need a decent bag to hold your swag; foraged fruits can get sweaty in a plastic food storage bag, especially when gathered under the glare of the midday sun. Your flimsy container may also come to a premature end when confronted with a thorny bush. A burlap or canvas tote bag is a good, durable option, especially when combined with a selection of plastic containers to separate your stash.

☑ *Tools*

A folding pruning knife can be useful for helping to persuade reluctant plants to give up their bounty. Likewise, a pair of long-nosed pruners may come in handy when delving deep for fruits or flowers borne on thorny bushes (see Gorse, *page 40*)

☑ *Protection*

Protection is key when foraging. Thornproof gloves are handy for preventing cuts and scratches, but they may be restrictive for nimble picking. In wintertime, a pair of fingerless gloves can provide cold weather protection while providing the necessary dexterity for your digits. A coat with capacious pockets will keep you warm and dry and also provide extra storage space for your foraged goods.

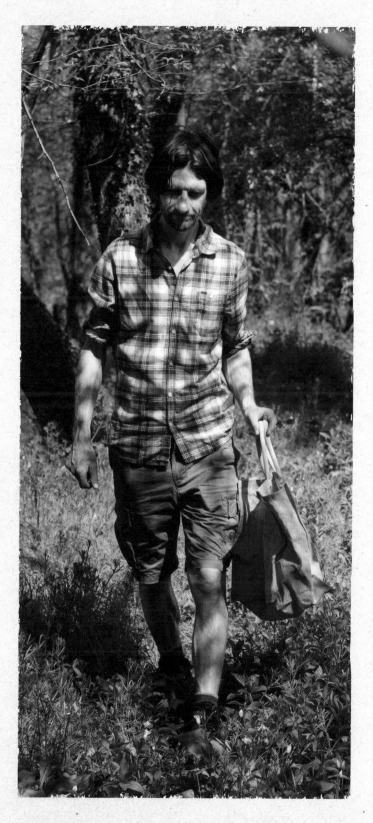

True Tea

The plants, flowers, berries, and roots mentioned in this book all make excellent brews but, for some folk, there is only one true tea—the drink made from the leaves of *Camellia sinensis*. If you're a "true" fan, you can learn about its origins, how to grow it yourself, and how to identify different types here.

THE TEA PLANT

CAMELLIA SINENSIS

The plant is thought to have originated in southwestern China (*sinensis* means "from China") and was used to make drinks for medicinal purposes in the third century AD. Its popularity spread during the Tang dynasty (AD 618–705) into neighboring Asian countries, reaching Europe sometime during the sixteenth century. Today, it's grown in around forty-five countries in a wide variety of climates, from tropical mountainous regions to the damp, weedy conditions of our plot here in the South West of England.

As with wines, the conditions in which the tea plant grows affect the taste and aroma of the final brew. These conditions—commonly known as "terroir"—include soil types, local weather conditions, and altitude. The most profound effect on flavor, however, is the way the tea leaves are processed after picking. Depending on the style of tea desired, tea makers will either macerate, roll, or tumble tea leaves to break down their cells before letting them oxidize (or "turn brown" to you and me). The longer the leaves oxidize, the darker and richer the tea will be. Green and white teas forgo the oxidization process, which results in a lighter, fresher brew.

For a lowdown on the various styles available, turn the page for our guide to tea types.

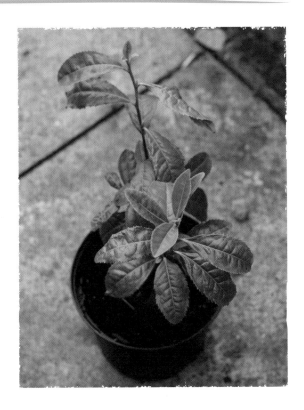

LEGENDARY TEA

According to Japanese legend, Bodhidharma, a fifth-century Buddhist monk, first created tea. Disgusted with himself for falling asleep while meditating, Bodhi sliced off his own eyelids and flung them to the ground. The first tea plant (complete with eyelid-shaped leaves) sprung from his discarded eyelids. Bodhi (in wide-eyed amazement) plucked the leaves and brewed the very first cup of tea.

1. GROW IT

You can grow a tea plant from seed, but germination can be a hit or miss affair. For ease, we suggest grabbing young plants, which are available from speciality nurseries and online garden retailers.

Tea plants like growing in acidic soil with good drainage, ideally in a location with part shade and shelter from the wind. Top-dress tea plants annually with shredded bark or well-rotted leaves (composted in a garbage bag with a few aeration holes for up to a year) and water well in the summer.

Although *Camellia sinensis* is frost hardy, container-grown plants can be susceptible to root damage caused by cold weather. To prevent a premature end to your tea plantation aspirations, swaddle the flowerpots with Bubble Wrap or a floating row cover in the winter.

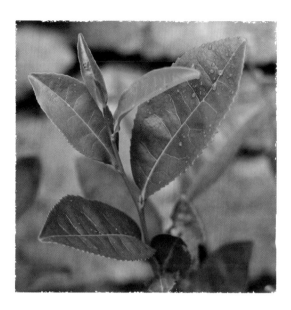

2. PICK IT

Tea plants take two to three years to reach maturity and will grow broad, bushy, and tall if left unpruned. To keep them manageable, and to aid easy picking, commercial tea plantations trim their bushes to waist height and flat to create a "plucking table." A tea plant is ready to be plucked when new, bright green growth (called the flush) starts to appear. For the best cup of tea, pluck the first two newly emerged leaves (including the bud) from the branch with a pincer action using your finger and thumb.

3. PREPARE IT

For Black Tea:

Bruise your plucked leaves using a mortar and pestle or something similar. Spread out the bruised leaves in a single layer and let them air dry for a couple of days. Put the leaves onto a baking sheet in an oven for 20 minutes at 210°F before storing them in an airtight container.

For Green Tea:

Put your leaves into a colander and steam them over a saucepan of boiling water for 2–3 minutes. When cool, roll the leaves into long log shapes, then let dry in a warm place until crispy. Store your leaves in an airtight container.

HOW TO TAKE A CUTTING

If you want to increase your tea plant collection for minimum cash outlay, try propagating a cutting, snipped from your plant in late summer.

Find a developing leaf that is growing on a green stem on your donor plant, and cut the stem diagonally with a sharp knife about a finger's width above the leaf joint and two to three fingers below.

Plunge the cutting into a small flowerpot filled with a decent potting mix and keep somewhere warm but out of direct sunlight. Make sure the plant gets a light spray of water daily.

When your plant reaches a height of 8–12 inches, you need to harden it off over the course of three weeks to prepare it for outdoor life. To do this, in the first week, leave your plant outdoors, covered with garden fleece and bring indoors at night. In week two, leave it outside, minus the garden fleece, but bring indoors at night. In week three, leave it outside during the day and cover with garden fleece at night.

A Guide to Tea Types

**Below we've listed the most popular types of tea made from
Camellia sinensis to help you identify them with ease.**

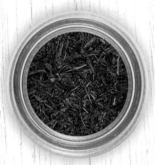

GREEN TEA

The most favored tea style in Asia. *Camellia sinensis*
leaves are plucked and heated—either by pan firing
or steaming—to prevent the leaves from oxidizing.
This process helps retain the tea's verdant color and
grassy, herbaceous flavors.

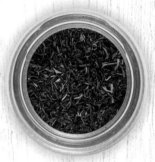

WHITE TEA

White tea is the result of a long, gentle process where
leaves (and sometimes unopened buds) wither for a
couple of days before being baked at a low heat. The tea
doesn't undergo any rolling or oxidization, which gives
it a light, delicate flavor. White tea gets its name from
the tiny white hairs* that cover the tips.

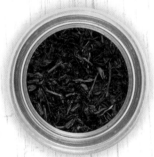

OOLONG TEA

To produce oolong tea, mature leaves are withered
in sunlight before being bruised to help release the
flavors prior to undergoing a partial oxidization.
Oolong tea is then either rolled into long leaves
or formed into tadpolelike shapes. The taste of
oolong can range from a fruity sweetness to herbal
and savory.

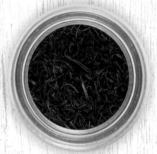

BLACK TEA

The ubiquitous tea bag tea widely favored for its full-
bodied flavor and high caffeine content. Leaves are
picked and bruised before undergoing full oxidization,
turning them black. Heat is then applied to stop the
oxidization, and the tea is graded for quality.

** Naming it "hairy tea" would have been a more difficult
product to market.*

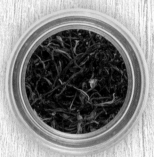

YELLOW TEA

Yellow tea is a rare, fragrant beast, made from the young buds taken from tea plants grown in select areas of China. Leaves are steamed so they oxidize slowly, which results in a straw-colored brew with a smooth, mellow taste.

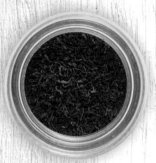

PU'ER TEA

This tea is the leafy equivalent of an aged whiskey. It's made from the large-leaf subspecies *Camellia sinensis* var. *assamica*, grown in Yunnan Province, southwestern China, which is fermented with a special bacterium, then pressed into cake shapes and aged. Because the tea is in a constant state of flux, no two teas will taste the same.

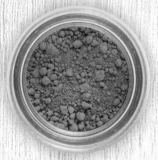

MATCHA TEA

Tea destined to be turned into matcha is shade-grown for three to four weeks before harvest, which stimulates chlorophyll production, hence the tea's bright green hue. In the matcha-making process, leaves' veins and stems are painstakingly removed before being ground into a fine powder, which results in a concentrated, caffeine-packed brew.

FLAVORED TEA

Adding flavoring was once used as a way to disguise poor-quality black teas—much like those grocery store cheeses that come in strange flavors (and a few fruit-flavored liquors, for that matter). Perhaps the most popular example is Earl Grey, which is flavored with bergamot oil. Lapsang souchong gets its smoky flavor by drying leaves over pinewood fires.

Milk

There was a time, in our youth, when milk was simply defined by the amount of cream it contained. But in these more health- and environmentally conscious times, not only is there a greater choice of dairy milk products around, but there's a bandwagon loaded with dairy-free milk alternatives that is rolling to a grocery store near you.

While many of the drinks made from nuts, grains, and seeds bear only a passing resemblance to the taste of anything a cow might produce, plenty of them are perfectly effective in a cup of tea, providing some of the whitening, texture-smoothing, and flavor-softening properties that would traditionally be performed by milk.

If you're new to plant-base milk alternatives, you should try a few different types to find the one that best suits your preferred drinks. For example, we reckon almond milk works well in a cup of chai; we count on coconut milk for the most wonderful turmeric latte; but when it comes to black tea, oat milk wins hands down.

Another great thing about milk alternatives is that you can even make some of them yourself, which (unless you're in charge of a dairy herd) is not something you can say about milk produced by a cow.

OAT MILK

For this recipe you'll need to get hold of some rolled oats. You can invest in an elaborate rolling machine that will mill and roll your own, home-grown oats (see *page 82*), but to be honest it's far easier to source some from the shops.

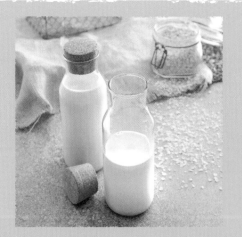

Makes: 4 cups
1 cup rolled oats
4 cups water
A pinch of salt
½ teaspoon vanilla extract and 1–2 teaspoons honey or maple syrup (optional, see right)

1 Pour the oats into a large bowl and cover with water, then set aside and let soak for 15–20 minutes.

2 Pour the wet oats into a strainer, rinse under cold water, and transfer to a food processor.

3 Add the water and salt, and the vanilla extract, honey or maple syrup (if using), then blend on full power for 1–2 minutes.

4 Finally, strain the oaty mixture through a strainer and chill before serving.

HAZELNUT MILK

You can apply the method given here for hazelnut milk to pretty much any kind of nut-base milk, but hazelnuts are easily foraged near us, so it's them we turn to for our wild and milky drinks. Goes well with coffee, too.

Makes: 3 cups
1 cup shelled, raw hazelnuts
3 cups water
½ teaspoon vanilla extract and 1–2 teaspoons honey
  or maple syrup (optional, see below)

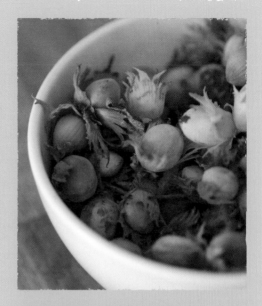

1 First, soak the nuts by putting them into a bowl and covering them with water. Refrigerate overnight (or for around 8 hours).

2 After soaking, pour off the liquid and rinse the nuts well under cold running water.*

3 Put the nuts into a blender with the water and blast until they have seemingly disappeared.

4 This liquid now needs straining. You can use specialty "nut milk bags," but a traditional fine straining cloth, such as cheesecloth, will work just as effectively. Make sure you squeeze the crushed nuts as hard as you can to extract every last drop of goodness. Add the vanilla extract and honey or maple syrup now (if using).

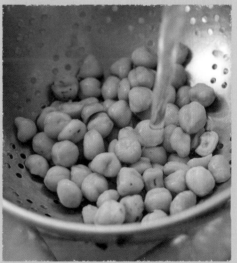

5 Store the liquid in a sealed bottle or jar and keep it in the refrigerator, where it will last for two days. The liquid separates if left alone, so make sure you shake your milky nut juice before each use.

OPTIONAL FLAVOR ENHANCERS

Although we find these simple nut and oat milk recipes perfectly acceptable for cups of tea, some people prefer extra flavor and sweetness to make them more dairylike when poured onto their morning cereal. If this sounds like you, try whisking in ½ teaspoon of vanilla extract and 1–2 teaspoons of honey or maple syrup.

* Some folk suggest peeling off the hazelnut's dark outer layer at this stage, but we don't think it is necessary. If you disagree and insist on a whiter milk, turn to page 171 for nut-blanching directions.

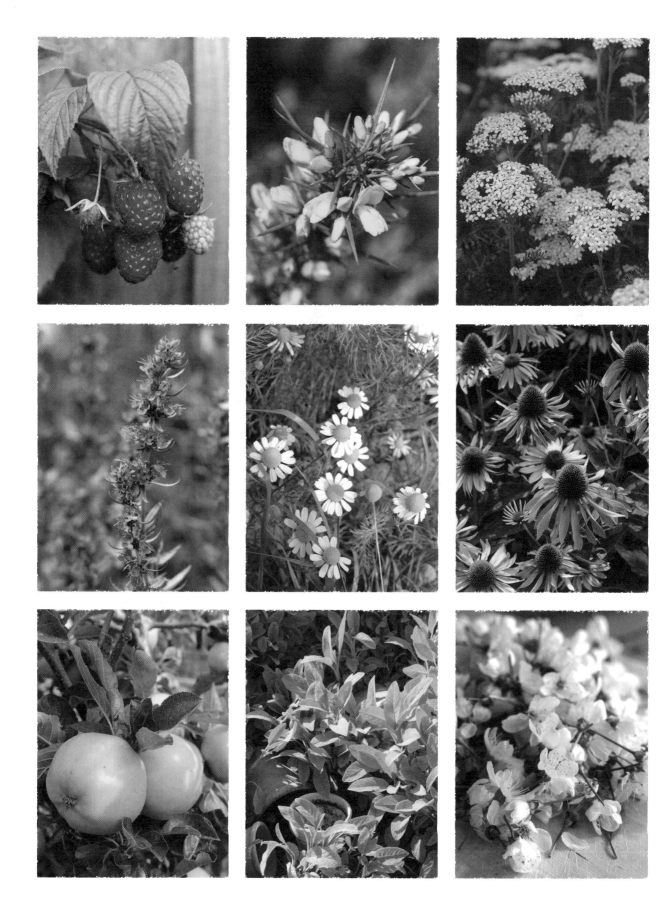

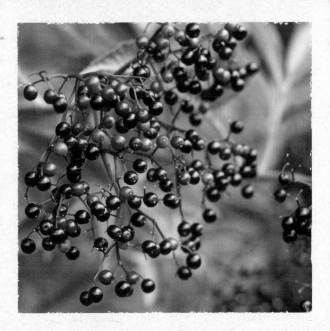

Top 40 Ingredients

Whether grown, foraged, or bought, these are our favorite choices for brewing a wild tea.

Blackberry

(Rubus fruticosus)

For us, the first foray into foraging was blackberry picking with our parents. We can still remember the excitement of picking these juicy jewels—for every berry nabbed, we'd shove at least five into our mouth. Blackberry bushes are prolific and easy to grow. You can brew both the berries and leaves, so load up in springtime when the fresh leaves start to appear, and then in late summer enjoy the bountiful berry bonus.

FORAGE IT

Wild blackberry bushes are common in the midwestern and eastern states and sometimes grow in warmer southern states, although the fruit will be small. According to folklore, the berries shouldn't be picked after Michaelmas (September 29), because the devil will either spit on them, pee on them, fondle them, or generally manhandle them. However, the spoiling of blackberry crops at this time is probably due to cool, damp weather instead of demonic intervention. Store the picked berries in a cool, dry place (they should last a couple of days) or freeze them for later. Pick the leaves and tips when they are young and fresh, before they develop tough spines on their undersides.

GROW IT

To all intents and purposes, there doesn't seem much point in cultivating your own blackberry bushes given their abundance in the countryside, but there are a few varieties available to grow in a yard or community garden that are worth considering. "Prime-Ark Freedom" will offer you wild-tasting fruit on a thornless plant, while the fruit of the "Osage" are sweet and flavorsome. For those who want a plant that can thrive in a container, consider the compact "Baby Cakes."

Most blackberry cultivars grow fruit on one-year old canes, so prune to the ground after harvesting the berries and tie or support any newly emerging canes the following spring.

BREW THE LEAVES

Blackberry leaves make fantastic tea and can be treated in much the same way as you would the leaves of *Camellia sinensis*. You can brew with fresh leaves but the best way of making blackberry leaf tea is to bruise the young leaves before letting them dry naturally so that they oxidize. The longer you leave them, the more intense flavor they will release. To make your cup of tea, crumble them up and steep 2–3 teaspoons in hot water for 5–10 minutes.

DID YOU KNOW?

During the American Civil War, blackberry tea was drunk by both Confederate and Union troops in an attempt to cure the rampant dysentery that plagued both sides. Ceasefires were often called so that soldiers could go out and forage for fruits to help stem the tide.

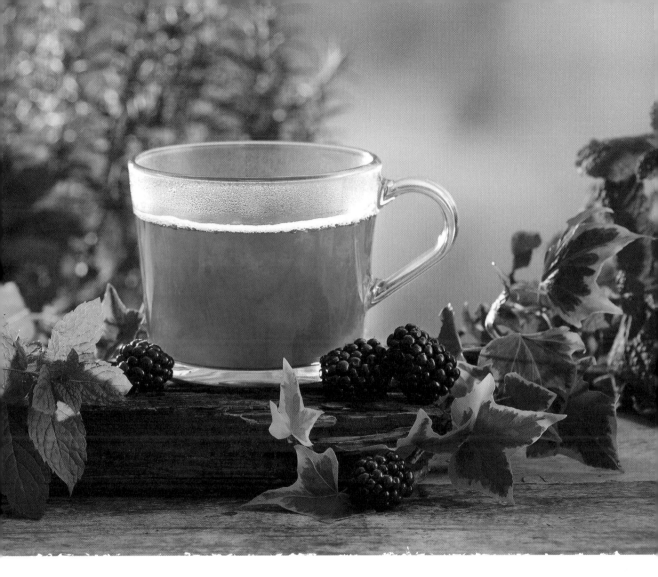

BREW THE BERRIES

Mash up a handful of blackberries,*
push the resulting mush through
a strainer, and let the syrup that is
released rest for a couple of hours on
a warm windowsill to steep. Pour the
mixture into a mug and top off with
hot water. Enjoy.

For a nice icy summertime treat,
head on over to *page 172* and try our
Blackberry Frappé recipe.

HEALTH BENEFITS

Blackberries pack plenty of fiber and
contain decent amounts of vitamin C
and vitamin K (vitamins that are
commonly found in green leaves),
which are an essential aid to the
blood-clotting process that heals
wounds. Blackberry leaf tea is also
said to be an effective cure for
acute diarrhea.

BLEND IT

Delve farther into the bushes and
try mixing the berry juice with its
countryside cousin elderberry for a
dark and fruity brew. Use the leaves
instead of green tea in healthy,
caffeine-free blends.

** Blackberries also bring
an autumnal, deep red
hue to infusions that
looks instantly healthy.
(The ivy in the picture
above is purely for
photogenic purposes —
its poisonous leaves
are most definitely not
healthy.)*

Black Currant

(Ribes nigrum)

The black currant is one of the most versatile homegrown ingredients in the tea maker's caddy—both its fruit and leaves are suitable for brewing. The leaves are full of tannin that gives a robustness similar to black tea. Used on its own, as a double act or blended with other ingredients, black currant rewards the drinker with a healthy tea full of tart curranty goodness.

GROW IT

If you live in a state where black currants are not banned (see facing page), they are one of the easiest soft fruit bushes to grow and are even suitable for containers. They're sold as "bare root stock" (the sticks have exposed roots) or in containers, and should be planted outside during their dormant period between November and March. Before planting, soak the roots well, then dig a large hole (around twice the diameter and depth of the roots when spread out), fill halfway with compost or manure, sink in the sticks, and fill with more compost. The dormant period is also the time to prune your currant bushes. Because the fruit is more bountiful on younger branches, it's the old ones that should be removed, along with any that are weak or damaged.

There are a few black currant cultivars to choose from, but "Consort" is one of the reliable ones.

BERRY HYBRIDS

Botanists like to experiment with berries, including black currants, and have come up with a number of hybrids. Here are five curranty couplings that can give your teas a twist.

Jostaberry

This cross between a black currant and gooseberry produces dark berries that start out dominated by the tart flavor of a gooseberry before taking on more of a black currant flavor as they mature.

Loganberry, Tayberry, and Tummelberry

Three different fruits, each the result of crossing blackberries with raspberries, and all coming in various shades of red.

Boysenberry

This sees the blackberry crossed again with one of its own offspring, the loganberry, to produce a sweeter kind of blackberry.

Silvanberry

An Australian creation, this is a cross between a boysenberry and a marionberry (a blackberry cultivar). It's essentially a blackberry.

Chuckleberry

This fruit with a silly name is a mongrel of the berry world, being a cross between a red currant, gooseberry, and jostaberry (see above). It grows like a black currant and is a high-yielding plant.

BREW THE BERRIES

The berries make an excellent rich and fruity tea with a distinctive tartness. To make, crush around 15 fresh berries by pressing them against the inside of a mug with a teaspoon (or for those who like getting messy with purple stains, a pinch between finger and thumb also works) before adding enough boiling water to fill the mug to the top. Let the berries steep for as long as possible for maximum flavor. You can also use dried or frozen fruits.

BREW THE LEAVES

The leaves share some of the flavors of the fruit, along with a fresh "greenness," and are packed with tannin, which will give your tea a bite. You'll need around 10 medium fresh leaves per cup. Crush them before adding the boiling water and remove after 4–5 minutes to prevent the tannins from taking over. They also work well dried; 1–2 teaspoons are enough for a brew.

HEALTH BENEFITS

Black currants are packed full of vitamin C, making the tea one of the healthiest you can brew. They have also been referred to as "gout berries," due to their ability to regulate the uric acid levels in the body that are responsible for gout and joint pains.

BLEND IT

The berries combine well with other fruits, and experimenters can have fun introducing them to a few fragrant flowers, such as rose or lavender. The leaves are great at adding a depth of flavor and bite to other ingredients— try a pinch in a mug of mint tea to give it a currant punch.

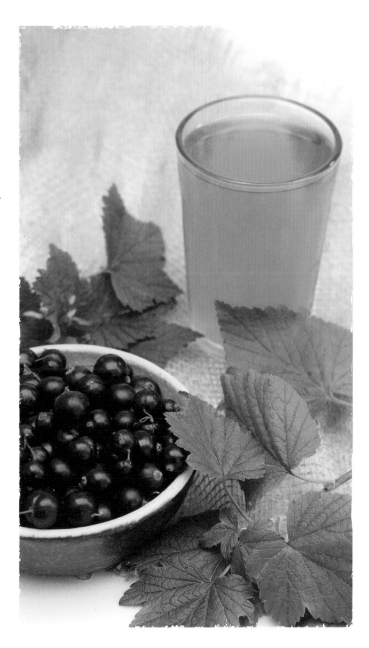

DID YOU KNOW?

It is illegal to grow black currants in a number of American states, because the plants can transmit the disease white pine blister rust, which damages native forests. Before you buy a plant, make sure there isn't a ban in your state.

Raspberry

(Rubus idaeus)

This beloved bringer of small ruddy fruits grows prolifically in our community garden, despite occupying the site of our longest running battle with weeds. Due to a sloppy mulching policy, in the summer the raspberry patch is overrun with bindweed, a plant-strangling perennial whose sole aim seems to be to pull down the berry-bearing canes and ruin our crop. Untangling the raspberries is a tedious but necessary task, so our bushes can provide us with both fruit for jams and desserts and terrific tannic leaves that are perfect for turning into tea.

GROW IT

Raspberries favor rich, well-drained, slightly acidic soil, preferably in a nice, sunny spot that is sheltered from strong winds. Plant them outside between September and March, when the canes are dormant. Dig some well-rotted manure into your chosen planting site and plant in rows, with each plant about 2 feet apart. There are two types of raspberry: summer fruiting and fall fruiting. Summer-fruiting plants are usually trained up a frame or post and wire support, but fall-fruiting plants can be left to their own devices. These are also the best bet for growing in a patio container.

To keep your plants healthy and productive, pruning is essential. If you have fall-fruiting canes, chop them all down in winter. Summer-fruiting canes need a little more care, so make sure you cut down the canes after they fruit (the woody ones), but leave the newer, greener canes so that they can produce fruit the following season. If you plan to grow both types, it's a good idea to plant them apart. The spreading nature of the runners means that the two types will soon intermingle if planted too close, causing extreme pruning confusion.

Your raspberry patch will benefit from a drop of fertilizer in early spring. Mulching around the base with well-rotted manure will also help keep pesky weeds at bay. If you treat them well, your raspberries will reward you with ten or more years of fruity pleasure.

BREW IT

To make the best raspberry leaf tea, pluck the youngest leaves from the stems and let dry. Use 1–2 teaspoons per cup and let infuse in a cup full of boiling water for 5–10 minutes. For added fruitiness, try drying out a few raspberry fruits (best done in a dehydrator) and drop them into your cup along with the leafy mix.

DID YOU KNOW?

Raspberries hail from the same genus (*Rubus*) and family (Rosaceae) as the blackberry, but what distinguishes the two is the stem (or torus). When you pick a blackberry, the stem stays with the fruit, while the raspberry leaves its stem behind, clinging to the plant.

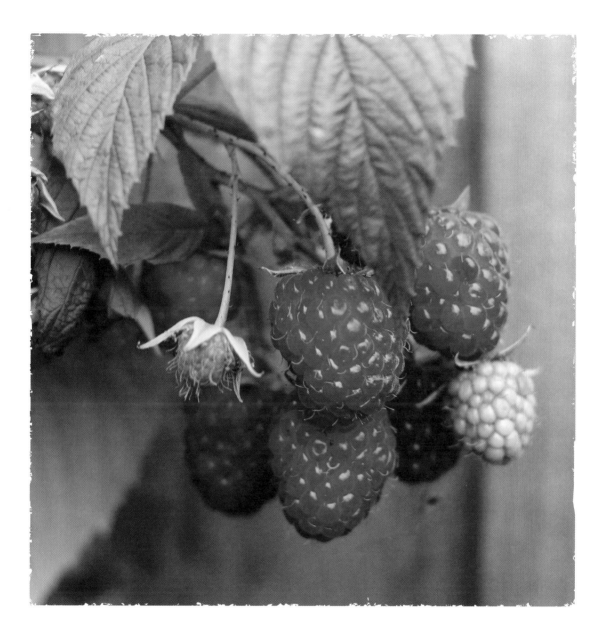

HEALTH BENEFITS

Raspberry leaf tea is sometimes taken by pregnant women, because it is believed to tone the uterus in preparation for the rigors of labor. In contrast, raspberry fruit tea tends to be taken purely for pleasure, but the fruit does contain decent amounts of anthocyanins, which are linked to a wide variety of health claims, including cancer prevention and the slowing of dementia symptoms.

BLEND IT

Try combining raspberry leaves with blackberry leaves, adding a twist of lemon for good measure. Raspberry and peppermint also make a tasty pairing, and the fruit makes a tart addition to both sun teas and fruit teas.

Spruce and Pine

(Picea and Pinus)

As spring turns to summer, the bright green new growth of spruce and pine tips emerge from their papery cases. They possess the freshest, cleanest essence of the forest, which produces one of the best-smelling teas around. Those tips are also packed with vitamin C, adding a healthy boost to its olfactory excellence.

FORAGE IT

Spruce (*Picea*) and pine (*Pinus*) tips first appear in late spring—soft, feathery, and almost glowing with vibrant green. The cultivars differ in looks and flavor, so hunt around to decide on your favorite. Also, check what you're picking, because similar-looking plants (notably yew) are poisonous. The tips pinch off easily, but don't get carried away by taking too many from one tree or you'll deprive it of the chance to fully grow.

GROW IT

If you want to plant a spruce or pine tree in the yard, then wait until December and get a container-grown Christmas tree (first checking with the grower that it hasn't been treated with chemicals, if you'll be consuming any of it). You should be able to nurse it through to spring with a little care. The popular Norway spruce is an excellent choice for tea making.

BREW IT

A small handful of tips (about 15 average tips) steeped in boiled water is enough for a cup of fresh tea, which is so popular in Sweden that it has its own name: *tallstrunt*. Tips are freezable and they also dry well, with 1 large teaspoon being enough for a brew. Older needles can be used to make tea, but they start to become more bitter and take on astringent flavors reminiscent of floor cleaning products, which is clearly not ideal.

HEALTH BENEFITS

Spruce and pine tips are so full of vitamin C that historically they were packed onto ocean-going vessels to help prevent scurvy among the crew. These days, people use them to treat a common cold. However, these are also ingredients with heavy cautions attached, and they should not be taken in large doses or by anyone who is pregnant or breastfeeding.

BLEND IT

The fresh lemony flavors of spruce and pine make them an interesting alternative to the lemon-tasting ingredients lemon verbena and lemongrass. They also make a good addition to a simple cup of green tea.

DID YOU KNOW?

Spruce and pine get their lemon flavors from limonene, one of several chemical compounds known as terpenes that are also found in citrus fruit. Pinene is another terpene present and is responsible for those piny flavors. Both compounds are used in cleaning products.

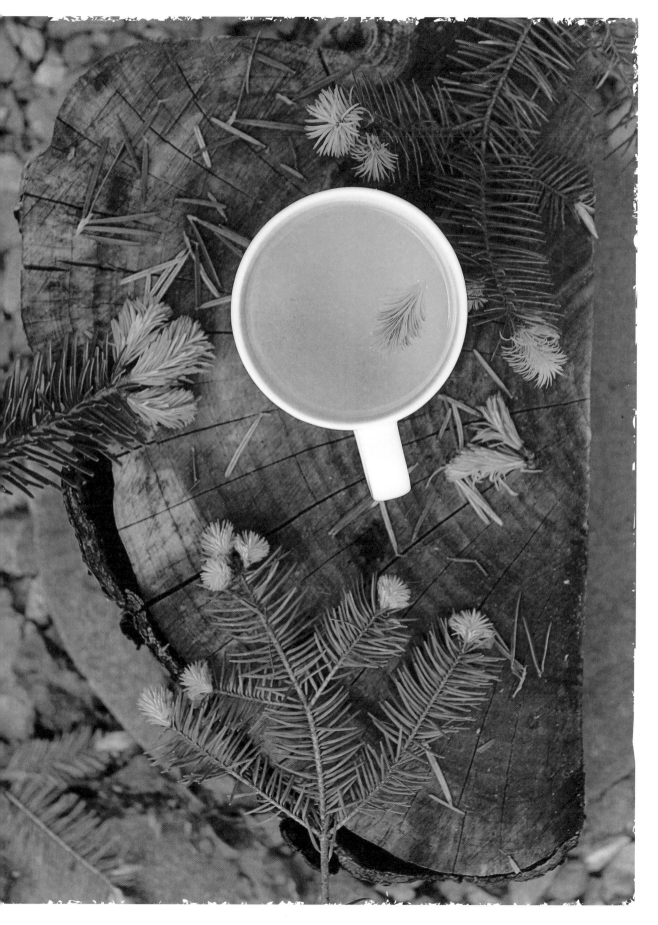

Hops
(*Humulus lupulus*)

Hops are best known for their use in beer, with cultivars producing a wide range of flavors, including citrus fruit, currant, and pine, and also imparting that all-important bitterness. These attributes contribute to an excellent, soothing cup of tea. It's the flowers (or cones) of the hop plant that contain the essential flavoring oils and they also make an attractive addition to the yard—particularly if, like us, you've got an untidy brewing shed for the plants to ramble over and hide.

FORAGE IT

We often find wild hops rambling through hedges. The plants are most easily seen when the hop cones start to form on the vines, which happens from midsummer onward. Hops need to be picked at their prime for best results—the box (right) tells you all you need to know.

GROW IT

Although you can grow hops from seed, by far the best option is growing them from bare root stems called rhizomes. Plant them in deep, well-drained soil in early spring. Hops grown commercially are typically trained to grow up tall trellises, which can reach heights of 25 feet. A popular hop cultivar is "Cascade," which is not only resistant to disease but will also provide plenty of hop cones for your brewing endeavors.

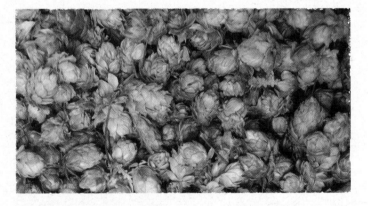

WHEN TO PICK YOUR HOPS

Most hops will be ready to harvest toward the end of summer. As the hops swell, they will take on a vibrant, fresh green color.

When ready, the vividness will begin to fade and you'll start to see some browning around the edges. Hops that are ready will feel dry and papery—gently rub them between finger and thumb and the petals will probably break off and your digits will feel sticky and oily.

Break up a cone and at the bottom of the petals you'll see the powdery yellow lupulin dotted around. It contains the all-important hop acids and essential oils that impart the flavor.

If you're still unsure, then wait a little longer—for brewing purposes, an overripe hop is better than an underripe hop.

BREW IT

Most brewers of beer will create a "tea" to help them predict the way a finished beer will taste (see *page 150*), and you can use the same method to produce a hot tasty beverage. We recommend using hops that are low in alpha acids (which determine the bitterness of the hop) such as "Williamette," because those with high alphas will make your tea unpleasantly bitter.

To brew a hot hoppy cup of tea, simply toss 4–5 fresh cones into a cup of boiling water and let infuse for 5–10 minutes before straining and serving.

HEALTH BENEFITS

The hop is a plant heralded for its sedative properties and, when steeped to make tea, you'll reap all of its snooze-giving goodness. Hops can also help with restlessness and irritability, and we can reliably confirm that these conditions are indeed relieved by a swift visit to a bar.

BLEND IT

Try mixing dried hops with nettles for an earthy, green-tinted brew. The zesty essence of lemon balm or lemon verbena also works well when combined (see *page 127*). Hops can also be used with other calm-inducing ingredients, such as those found in Sue's Hop to Bed Tea (see *page 126*).

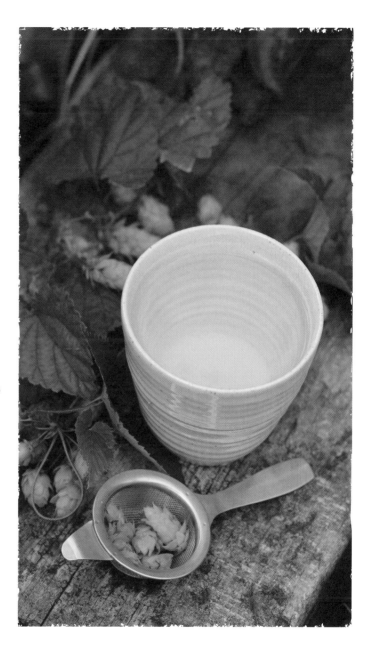

DID YOU KNOW?

The hops' habit of wrapping itself around surrounding vegetation led the Romans to believe that it could strangle and kill other plants. It was given the predatory name of "little wolf," which is a translation of the Latin genus name *Lupulus*.

Linden Flower

(*Tilia cordata*)

One of the most overlooked summer fragrances belongs to the linden, known in the UK as a lime tree*—perhaps because the blossom is mostly above nose height. But gather a handful of the delicate flowers, breathe in their aroma, and you will be rewarded with a wonderful, sweet perfume of ripe melon and honey. The resulting tea is popular in France, where it's known as *tilleul* and keeps Parisians in a calm, relaxed state of mind after a day stuck on the Boulevard Périphérique.

FORAGE IT

Linden trees can be old,** and grow most in the eastern states. The flowers speckle the trees in summer, as the days reach their maximum length, and are often covered with bees—its pollen is much appreciated by beekeepers for the tasty honey it produces. You should be able to gather enough blossoms at head height, but to maximize your picking potential, a chair or ladder will come in handy.

BREW IT

The leaves and even the bark of the linden tree can be used to make a variety of potions, but it's the flowers that make the best tea. You can use them fresh, but they are usually better when dried. The honey aroma remains after brewing and the flavor is clean and light, making a tea that is both calming and refreshing. Steep 1–2 teaspoons for 5–10 minutes. Sweet-toothed drinkers can stir in a teaspoon of honey.

HEALTH BENEFITS

Some people believe that linden flowers will ease colds and headaches as well as regenerate the skin, but linden flower tea is most often used to bring a sense of calm to the drinker, making it a good beverage during anxious moments or before heading off to bed (see *page 126*).

BLEND IT

Linden flower is most often blended with other sleep-inducing ingredients, such as chamomile and lavender.

DID YOU KNOW?

Marcel Proust, in his novel *In Search of Lost Time*, describes how a madeleine (a type of small cake) dipped in linden flower tea sets off a childhood memory and has led to the phrase "Proust's madeleine" being used as an expression for such memory triggers.

---

* *No relation to the citrus lime fruit, our tea-making blossom comes from the* Tilia *genus of trees.*

** *Westonbirt, The National Arboretum, in Gloucestershire, England, has a coppiced linden tree that is believed to be around 2,000 years old.*

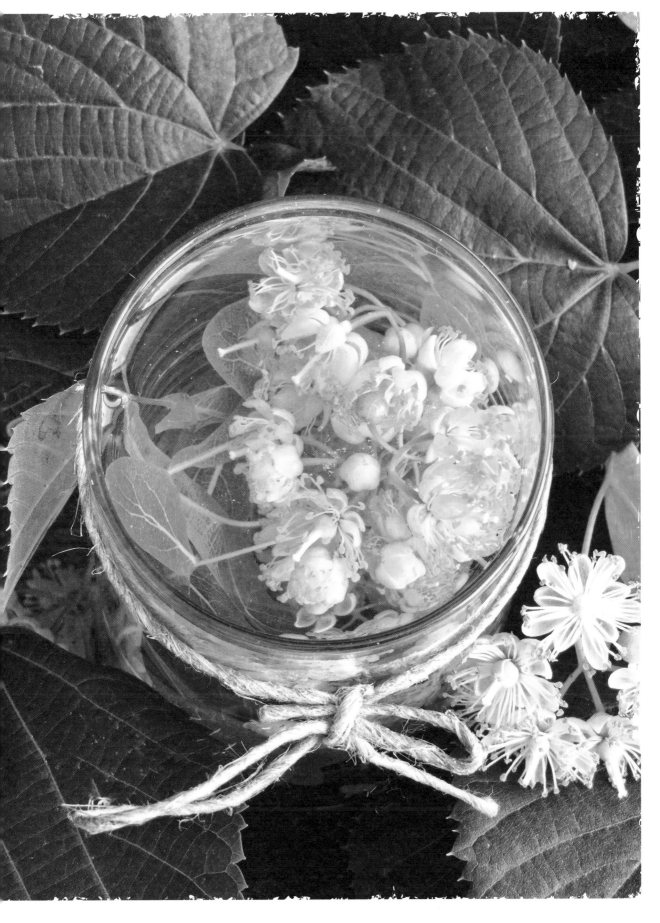

Gorse

(Ulex europaeus)

Gorse (also known as whin or furze) is a large, prickly member of the pea family, prized by foragers for its egg-yolk yellow flowers that can impart a distinctive coconut flavor to drinks and syrups. Its heady scent becomes more pungent in the heat of the sun, while the popping sounds of the seed heads may well punctuate a summer stroll through scrub. Gorse has been introduced to the east and west coasts, so with a little searching (and providing you like the distinctive flavor that the flowers impart) in these areas, you can add them to your tea mug.

FORAGE IT

With its bright yellow flower heads contrasting against the dark foliage, a gorse in bloom is easy to see. It flourishes in poor soil conditions and it is in these areas that you should look for them. Foraging for gorse flowers can be a tricky business thanks to the plants' prickly thorns. We suggest using a pair of long-nosed scissors and snipping the blooms directly into your chosen vessel.

GROW IT

Gorse is a great choice if you are looking to create an impenetrable barrier hedge to help keep out livestock* and intruders. However, it is considered an invasive species so if you choose to grow it in your yard, do so with care to avoid it spreading. You can grow gorse from seed, gathered on your foraging excursions. Soak seeds in water for 24 hours, then sow into trays, preferably under glass. Keep your newly planted gorse weed-free until the roots establish and give it a good pruning in early spring.

BREW IT

To make a tasty cup of tea, add 1 teaspoon of gorse flowers to a cup of boiling water and let them steep for 10 minutes before straining. Alternatively, let your brew cool and add ice and a slice of lemon for a subtle summertime sipper.

HEALTH BENEFITS

When scarlet fever was rife, children who caught the disease were often given an infusion of the flowers to ease symptoms. And while we don't necessarily endorse it as a toothpaste substitute, chewing a mouthful of gorse blossoms mixed with honey makes for a half-decent mouth cleanser after a night drinking beer.

BLEND IT

Try creating a Thai-inspired tea by blending your gorse flowers with a ¾-inch piece of lemongrass and ½ teaspoon of ginger.

DID YOU KNOW?

The gorse flower was once used as a soap substitute by combining it with clay. Presumably, first the thorns would have been carefully removed.

* *Disclaimer: During the eighteenth and nineteenth centuries, gorse was widely used as animal fodder, so you may well attract more hooved beasts than you repel.*

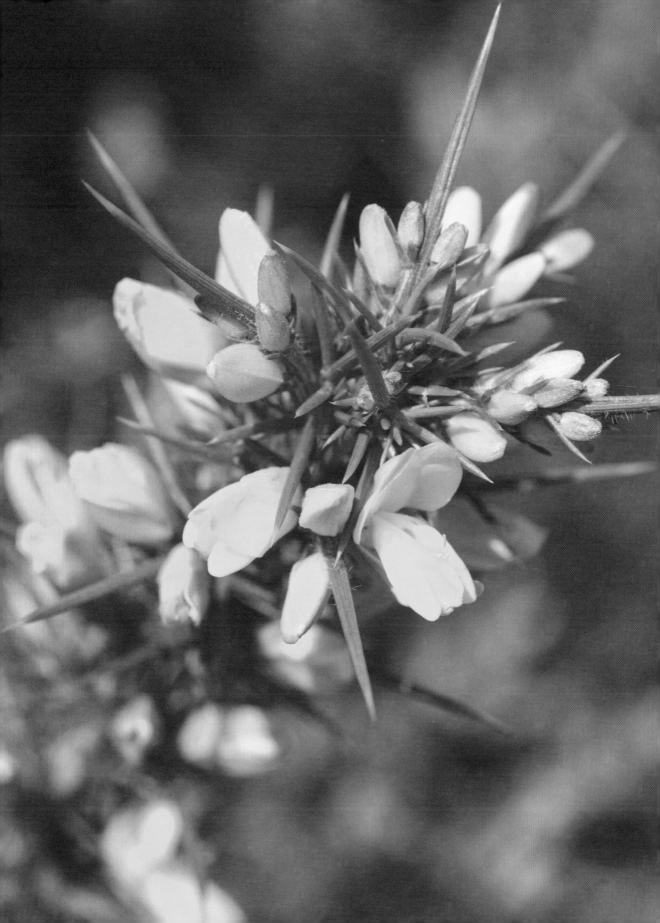

Hawthorn

(Crataegus monogyna)

The hawthorn (or May tree) has long been a forager's favorite. The young, emerging leaves* and berries can be eaten directly from the bush and have earned the nickname "bread and cheese" (despite tasting of neither bread nor cheese). Its nutty-flavor foliage is a tasty addition to salads, but the hawthorn excels when it comes to hot, steamy beverages. Leaves, flowers, berries—you can brew them all.

FORAGE IT

Like many plants destined for the teapot, the young leaves are the most flavorsome. The same applies to the flowers, which you should pick soon after they emerge. You'll have to wait a little longer for the berries to arrive, but be patient—underripe fruit will produce weak, tasteless tea, so ideally you'll want to hold back until it is nice and plump. To test whether your berries are ready for the pot, gently squeeze them; if the fleshy package gives a little, they're ready for the pot.

BREW THE FLOWERS AND LEAVES

Dunk a fresh sprig (leaves and flowers) into a cup of boiling water and let infuse for 5–10 minutes for a delicately flavored, green-hued brew. For a more intense hit, first dry the leaves,

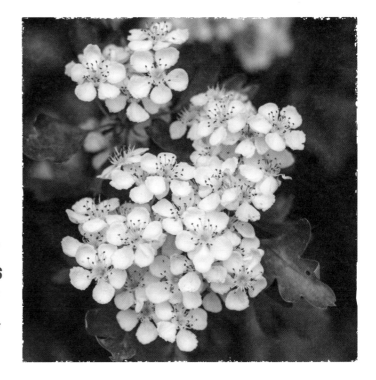

DID YOU KNOW?

The hawthorn is a plant shrouded in superstition. In folklore, it is believed to be a harbinger of death, not least because the pungent odor of the hawthorn flower reportedly smells like rotting flesh. In the poem "Whitsun," Sylvia Plath recalls picnicking among the "death stench of hawthorn." We'd argue that our tea has a more fragrant aroma.

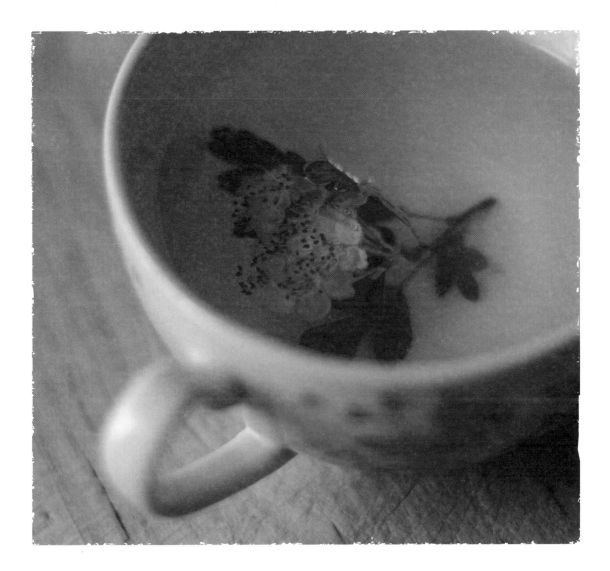

then coarsely chop them and use 1–2 teaspoons per cup.

BREW THE BERRIES

Wash your berry bounty, then slice them before drying, ideally in a dehydrator. Add 2 teaspoons per cup, pour on freshly boiled water, and let infuse for 10 minutes for a pleasant, slightly tannic, orange-hued brew.

HEALTH BENEFITS

Hawthorns have been used for centuries to lower blood pressure and improve circulation, and the fruit is a key player in traditional Chinese medicine. However, it is best to use hawthorn with caution— consuming vast quantities can have an adverse effect on the heart and cause palpitations. Regardless, you should be fine sipping a few cups of tea.

BLEND IT

You can try blending the berries with hawthorn's pal the rosehip (it can be found growing nearby) for a vitamin C-packed, health-giving brew.

* *Older leaves, like stale bread and cheese, are inedible.*

Elderberry

(Sambucus nigra)

Old countryside wisdom from England says summer starts with the arrival
of elderflowers and ends when the berries are ripe. We've endured a few lousy
summers that have started in mid-August and ended in torrential downpours
a couple of weeks later, but we get the general idea. Elderflowers are, of course,
synonymous with the making of elderflower champagne. If you can resist
using all of your gathered stash for this bubbly treat, try setting some aside
for a floral-forward cup of tea. In late August, return to the elderberry tree and
plunder its berries for pummeling into dark and funky brews.

FORAGE IT

If possible, collect your elderflowers
before noon, because as soon as the
midday sun starts to heat up the
flowers, they will start to give off a
heady smell similar to cat pee. Shake
and wash them well, because you'll
find a menagerie of insects lurking
among the flowers, the likes of which
are not necessarily conducive to a nice
brew. Pick the berries when they ripen
to a deep purple hue in late summer.
Be aware that the berries (and leaves,
stems, shoots, and roots) are toxic
until cooked, so don't be tempted to
have a nibble while you're out picking.

GROW IT

You shouldn't have much trouble
sourcing elderberries and flowers
in the wild, but if you want to grow
a pair of shrubs in your yard, we
suggest trying "York" with "Adams"
or "Nova." These ornamental shrubs
will take to most soil conditions and
will cross-pollinate for an increased
yield. Elderberry also grows easily from
cuttings—simply thrust a stick into
soil for a good chance it will take root.

BREW THE FLOWERS

Put 1 tablespoon dried elderflowers in
a cup and fill with boiling water. Let
steep for 5–10 minutes. Strain and
sweeten with honey to taste.

BREW THE BERRIES

Dried berries make a decent cup of
tea, but using fresh berries is a little
more involving. A tea brewed from
elderberries alone can be pretty tangy,
so it pays to add a few spices to make
it into a chai. Grab a fistful of fresh
elderberries, pound them into a paste,
then put it into a saucepan. Add
2 cardamom pods, ½ a cinnamon stick,
1 teaspoon of freshly grated ginger,
and 1¼ cups of water. Bring to a boil
and simmer for 10 minutes. Strain
into a mug and enjoy.

DID YOU KNOW?

It is thought that
flies are repelled
by the scent
of elderberry
leaves, so these
shrubs were often
planted outside
fly-frequented
buildings, such
as latrines, farm
buildings, and
slaughterhouses.

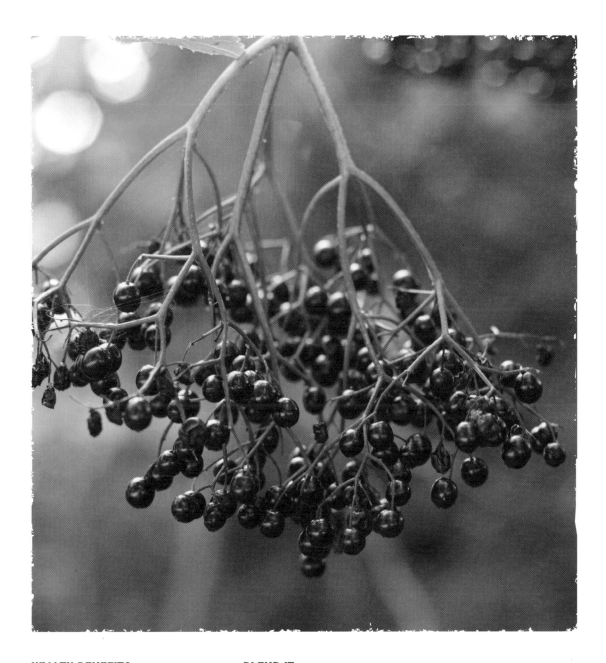

HEALTH BENEFITS

Elderflowers are thought to have antiseptic and anti-inflammatory properties and are often used in traditional medicine to help treat sinusitis and joint pains. Elderberries are a strong antioxidant and pack plenty of fiber.

BLEND IT

A brew made from elderflowers requires subtle flavor combinations— try it with raspberry leaves or rose petals, which are arguably at their best in a summery iced tea (see *page 158*). The bold berries of elder work well with other dark berries and the addition of spices.

Queen of the Meadow

(Filipendula ulmaria)

You'll find this wispy member of the rose family, which is also known as meadowsweet, growing in eastern and some midwestern states. The name "meadowsweet" is derived from the Anglo-Saxon word *medesweete*, because the plant was once used to make mead, a heady, honey-base booze renowned for bestowing fearful hangovers. Ironically, the plant contains salicin, a precursor to the drug aspirin, making it both a cause and a cure for a headache. Feeling a little fragile? A cup of queen of the meadow tea might be just the tonic.

FORAGE IT

Queen of the meadow is easy to find, thanks to the white frothy blooms billowing from tall reddish stems. Its sweet, almondlike scent is also a strong giveaway, which becomes more intense after picking—you'll certainly notice a pleasing aroma as the flowers sit drying on your kitchen window.

GROW IT

The plant prefers growing wild and free but will grow in a garden setting. However, queen of the meadow is considered invasive in some states, such as Missouri, so check before planting. It prefers full sun but will tolerate semi-shade. Plant it in rich, moist soil, mulch it with well-rotted manure, and cut back after flowering.

BREW IT

Queen of the meadow tea is taken more for its perceived health benefits than for taste, but we think there's a certain understated charm to its subtle, strawlike flavor. Add 1 teaspoon of dried flowers to a cup of boiling water, let infuse for 10 minutes, then strain before drinking.

BLEND IT

Queen of the meadow is not often used in blended brews due to its delicate nature, but you can try it in our Coastal Cup on *page 123*.

HEALTH BENEFITS

Along with helping to stem the misery of a throbbing head, queen of the meadow has traditionally been used as a digestive aid. The plant is also used as a cure for diarrhea and in the treatment of inflammatory diseases. It also contains salicylic acid, which is used in the production of aspirin, so be careful when drinking it and only do so in moderation. It should not be consumed during pregnancy and by anyone with an aspirin allergy. Folk who have asthma should also give this plant a wide berth.

DID YOU KNOW?

Queen of the meadow was used extensively in the Middle Ages as a strewing herb. Strewing herbs were sprinkled onto floors so that they would release a perfumed scent when crushed underfoot and mask unpleasant odors. In those days of open sewers, plagues, and a slack approach to personal hygiene, there would have been many odors to mask.

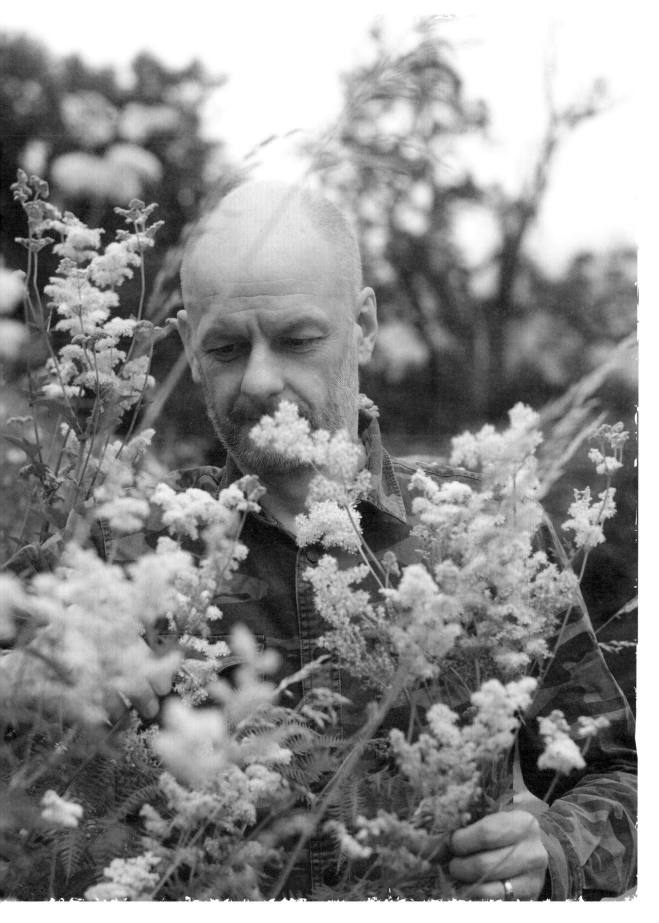

Hibiscus

(Hibiscus sabdariffa)

There are hundreds of species of hibiscus,* which belongs to the mallow family, but it is roselle (sometimes known as red sorell) that is widely cultivated for culinary use. Its tart, fruity flavors have been used in numerous drinks, preserves, sauces, syrups, and even pickles, where it quickly imparts its strong flavor and vivid red color to whatever it meets. A colorful essential for your tea caddy.

GROW IT

If you want to grow your own from seed, you will need to make small incisions into the hard coating and soak the seeds in warm water for 2 hours prior to planting. The plants then need careful nurturing, particularly in a cold and wet climate, and will bloom as summer fades to fall. This is all slightly too much work for us,** but thankfully dried roselle hibiscus is readily available.

BREW IT

It's actually the red calyces of hibiscus that are used for beverages (the parts that surround the bud before flowering—they're green on most plants, such as roses) and their tricky removal is another reason to go down the store-bought route. To make a tea, simply steep 1 teaspoon of dried calyces in hot water for 5 minutes and you'll be rewarded with a bright red liquid that has a tart, fruity flavor.

HEALTH BENEFITS

There has been recent research into hibiscus tea to determine if it can help lower blood pressure and cholesterol. Its effect on the former has shown more promising results thus far (but our natural skepticism means we'll wait for more convincing evidence).

BLEND IT

Hibiscus has such a fruity flavor that many commercial tea blends claiming to be made with fruit actually have hibiscus as their main ingredient. For home blending, it's great for adding to dried fruits and berries, particularly if you want to capitalize on its red color. It also works well in iced teas (see *page 149*) and adds a punchy flavor to floral blends.

---

* *Some folk claim all species are edible, but we can't find evidence that they've all been tested. Stick to Hibiscus sabdariffa.*

** *We once successfully germinated some seeds but the young plants perished while we were on vacation.*

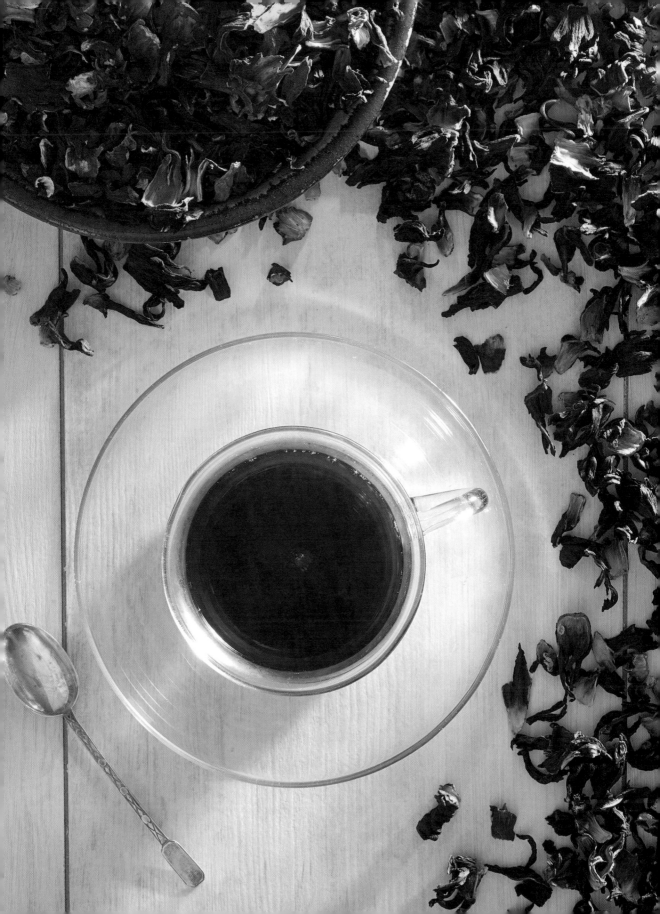

Yarrow

(Achillea millefolium)

We think yarrow is one of the most underappreciated wild plants around. Its masses of small white (and occasionally pink-tinged) flowers look as good in yards as they do in thickets, while its wispy, furry leaves make a superb cup of tea. Despite this, it doesn't seem to have caught on outside of the foraging fraternity, so head out into the fields and brew a cup—the yarrow appreciation club starts here.

FORAGE IT

Yarrow is common throughout North America, Europe, and, Asia, growing alongside roads, in meadows, on riverbanks, and just about anywhere else it's allowed to settle. It flowers in the summer and novice foragers should be careful to avoid confusion with similar looking white-flowering plants, particularly the deadly hemlock, so study its feathery leaves to help you to identify it correctly.

GROW IT

Other achillea cultivars are popular with gardeners, but yarrow is seen more as a weed. We think this harsh, finding it the most naturally attractive of the family, and we have gladly allowed it into our gardens (although its vast armies of tiny seed do have a habit of invading lawns). Insects love its flat-topped floral landing pads, which makes it an even more welcome member in our borders.

BREW IT

The leaves have a slight bitterness, which makes them a great addition to beers (but as with tea, you'll struggle to find it featured in many commercial brews). They're best used fresh for tea, producing a flavor similar to green tea—full of green vitality with an added earthiness. Flavor intensity can fluctuate, but 3–5 fresh leaves, depending on size, should be enough when steeped in a cup of hot water, or 1 teaspoon of dried leaves and flowers.

HEALTH BENEFITS

There is a huge list of mostly unsubstantiated health benefits attributed to yarrow—from curing fevers and healing wounds to treating hemorrhoids and skin conditions—but it should be used in moderation, because it can cause rashes in some cases, and it is toxic to cats, dogs, and horses.

BLEND IT

As with green tea, it goes well with lemon or mint.

DID YOU KNOW?

According to Greek mythology, Achilles used yarrow to heal his soldiers' wounds. The latin name *Achillea millefolium* is derived from the Greek words *achilleios*, which means "herb of Achilles," and *myriophyllon*, which translates as "countless leaves."

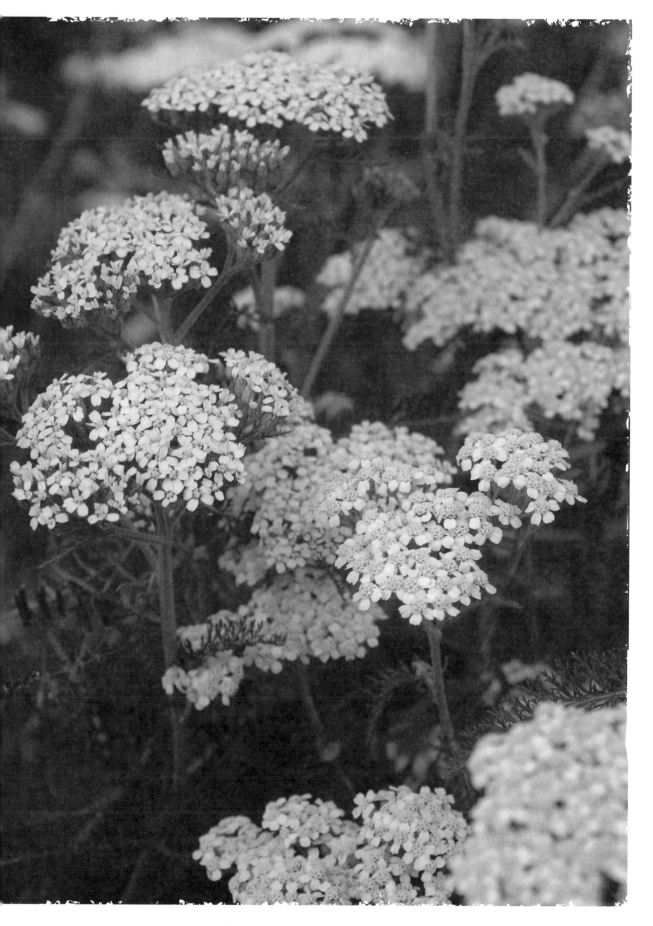

Mint

(Mentha)

If you grow one wild tea, make it mint. The herb is one of the easiest to grow and produces a constant supply of leaves from spring through to mid-fall, which can be used on their own or in a huge range of tea blends. Get yourself a container, stick it in the yard or on the windowsill, and treat yourself to a ready supply of instant refreshment.

GROW IT

Mint has a habit of rapidly spreading its roots, so confine it to flowerpots if you don't want it to take over your yard. The plants die back over winter and eagerly emerge as the spring warmth builds, increasing their coverage a little farther each year. Mint is also easy to cultivate from cuttings. Simply snip off a finger-length tip of stem just below a pair of leaves, remove the lower leaves, and stick the stem in a glass, filling it with water to below the leaves. Before long, roots will emerge and you can plant it in potting mix. If you find a plant you like, it's a great way to share the minty goodness with your friends.

BREW IT

Around 10 fresh leaves is enough for a cup, but you can pack as much of a minty punch as you want by adding more. Scrunch up the leaves to help release the flavor before infusing with hot water. Mint is also excellent dried with 1 teaspoon being enough for a mug.

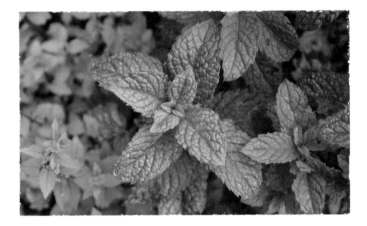

HEALTH BENEFITS

Besides freshening breath (see Morning After the Night before Tea, *page 126*) mint's main medical claims relate to the stomach. It can aid digestion and soothe pains, particularly when overeating is responsible (see *page 126*).

BLEND IT

Although mint can be a dominant flavor, it works well with most things, so put on your experimental hat and dream up some ingenious new combinations. For the traditional Moroccan Mint Tea see *page 137*.

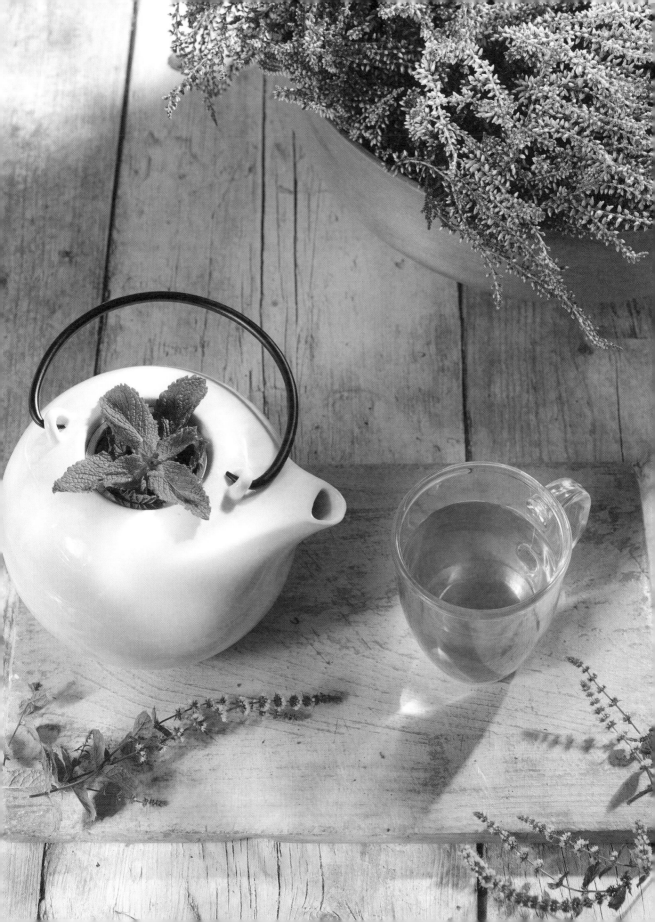

FIVE MINT VARIETIES

Wander around a well-stocked garden center or nursery and you'll probably find a wide range of mints, many claiming to have tastes similar to other foods (such as pineapple mint, chocolate mint, or banana mint). For tea makers, here are five mints we think it's worth getting to know:

Spearmint

Also known as common mint, garden mint, mackerel mint, and sage of Bethlehem, this is the classic upright, bushy mint with vivid green, tooth-edge leaves and sweet menthol flavors that make it great for all culinary uses, including teas.

Peppermint

A hybrid of spearmint and water mint, this herb is bolstered with extra menthol (40 percent compared to less than 1 percent in spearmint). Besides the increased minty flavor, it's also spicier and is often the preferred choice in commercially dried teas.

Moroccan mint

Moroccan mint is a type of spearmint with more compact leaves. Obviously, it's a good choice for Moroccan mint tea.

Apple mint

One of our favorite mints for the yard, this variety grows tall, has light green fluffy leaves, and is also known as tickle mint. It has a deliciously sweet and fruity minty flavor.

Ginger mint

Also known as Scotch mint, this is a cross between spearmint and corn mint. It's often seen showing off stripes on its leaves and has a subtle spicy warmth to its flavor.

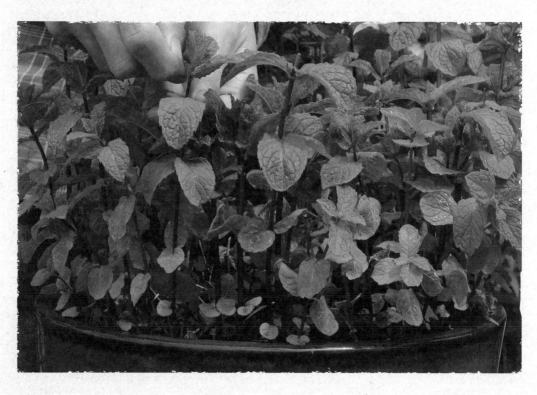

Dandelion

(Taraxacum officinale)

For us, the dandelion is a welcome sight in spring, with its showy yellow flower heads rising up from winter slumber to greet the sun. The name "dandelion" is believed to stem from the similarity between the plant's jagged leaves and the teeth of a lion. Likewise, the dandelion's long, incisor-like tap roots look equally toothy when dug out and extracted from the soil. Many folk consider it a weed, but we positively welcome it into our yard—you can make tasty tea and a great cup of coffee from this tenacious, lawn-loving plant.

FORAGE IT

Forage your dandelions in springtime for tender shoots and newly emerged flowers. Hunting in fall is best for gathering large, pendulous roots to turn into coffee. Dig down deep with a trowel to maximize your haul.

GROW IT

Gardeners with a slack approach to lawn care will undoubtedly have a limitless supply of dandelions to call on, but if you do feel the need to cultivate them, dig and chop up pieces of root, place them on the surface of a flowerpot filled with potting mix, and cover with a fine layer of potting mix. If you develop an insatiable appetite for dandelion, you can cultivate them into huge Frankensteinian specimens. Mulch the plants copiously with well-rotted manure and hill up the lower leaves to stimulate growth. Think Audrey II from *Little Shop of Horrors*, but with a smiley yellow face.

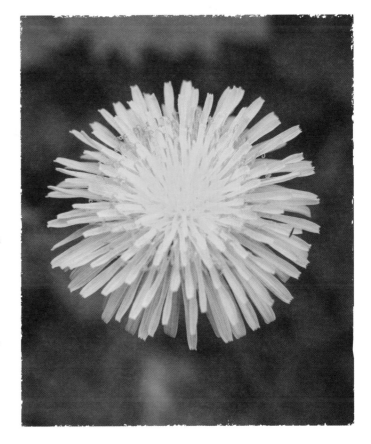

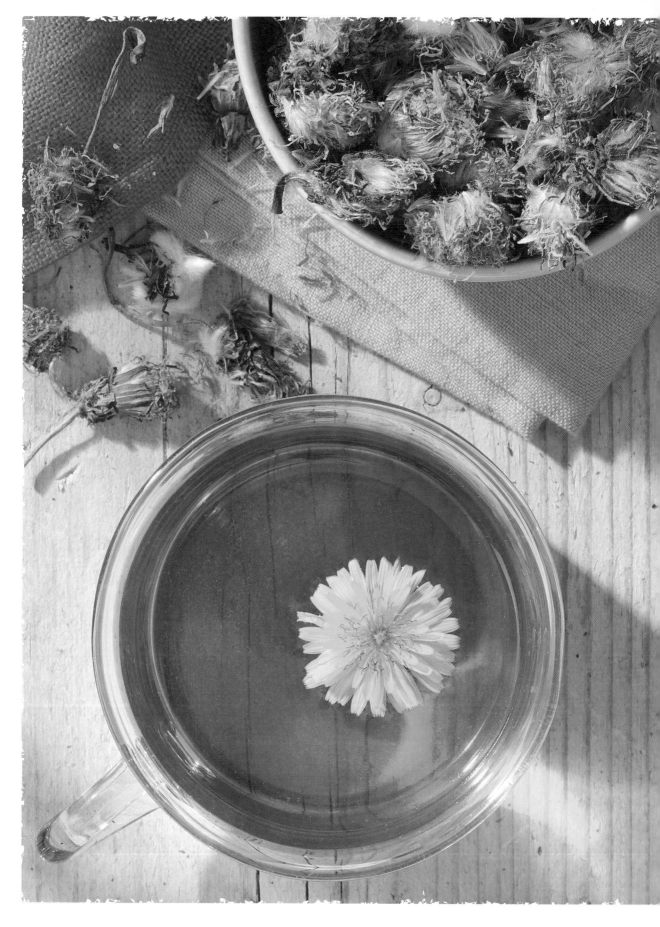

BREW IT

Pluck the petals from a handful of flower heads and steep in boiling water for 5–10 minutes. For a speedier dandelion fix, you can dunk whole flower heads into your mug, but expect a slightly bitter beverage. For a leafy brew, gather and dry young dandelion leaves. Use 1 teaspoon per cup and let infuse for 5 minutes. The undisputed king of dandelion brews can be made from the root. Head on over to *page 168* for our Dandelion Coffee recipe.

HEALTH BENEFITS

According to the law of the school playground, the merest flick from a dandelion will cause the unlucky recipient to wet the bed. This childish superstition is not without merit, because in traditional medicine, dandelions are considered a useful diuretic and are also used for treating heart problems, high blood pressure, and diseases of the liver and kidney. Flowers are also taken by folk who have a cold.

BLEND IT

You'll see dandelion leaves and flowers cropping up in numerous commercially available, healthy blends. We've combined them with other "weeds" for our Wild Garden Tea (see *page 123*).

DID YOU KNOW?

The dandelion's pant-wetting potential has blessed it with many regional nicknames. Our favorites include: **piss-i-beds** (England), *pissenlit* (France), and **bumpipes (Scotland).**

SOME SURPRISING USES FOR DANDELIONS

Drink!

As well as making fine hot beverages, dandelions can also be used in making booze. In times of hop shortages, brewers would often turn to dandelion leaves to provide bittering and flavor, while makers of country wines have long claimed that the flowers produce one of the finest tipples.

Eat!

Most of the dandelion is edible, from the roots to the flowers, but the milky stalks are off-limits, because they contain toxins that cause illness in some people.* Its young leaves are perhaps the most appetizing—in fact, you'll find them tucked among chervil, endives, and a variety of lettuce leaves in mesclun, a tasty and tender green salad that hails from Provence.

Drive!

One of the most unusual uses of dandelions is currently being explored by German tire manufacturer Continental. Dandelion roots contain a natural rubber and the company hopes that it will provide a sustainable alternative to the current, environmentally unfriendly components.

* *We have heard of dandelion stalk juice being squirted onto warts in the hope they miraculously disappear, but along with other wart "cures," such as banana peel, potatoes, and garlic, success seems unlikely.*

Rosemary

(Salvia rosmarinus)

Rosemary is an herb with a unique aroma and flavor. We might describe it as being piny, savory, slightly bitter, a touch peppery, and with even a hint of lemony sharpness but, whatever that flavor, it's great in drinks. As well as dunking it in hot water for tea, of course, we use it frequently in beer and as a cocktail garnish.

GROW IT

Rosemary is native to warmer regions of the world—the Mediterranean and Asia—and grows in parts of North America, but it's fairly hardy and only fails in extremely cold spots. Besides warmth, its main requirement is drainage, so if you have heavy soil, dig in some horticultural vermiculite before planting. It's an evergreen plant and can be regularly trimmed in spring and summer, with new growth constantly replenishing the plant. Go easy in winter, however, because it will need its strength to survive the cold instead of producing new shoots.

BREW IT

Rosemary's flavor intensity can vary throughout the year, but generally 2 freshly plucked sprigs are ample for a cup of tea. We like the instant freshness of newly picked sprigs, but it also dries well—use 1 teaspoon per cup of boiling water. If you're looking to impress, sprinkle a few of its soft purple flowers onto the water's surface.

HEALTH BENEFITS

Rosemary is noted for its ability to improve "prospective memory" (remembering to do something in the future, such as perhaps returning this book to the library) with the hope being that it may one day help prevent dementia. There are several other medicinal claims made about the herb, but we've forgotten what they are.

BLEND IT

Besides other herbs, we think it pairs well with tart and citrusy flavors, such as hibiscus and orange.

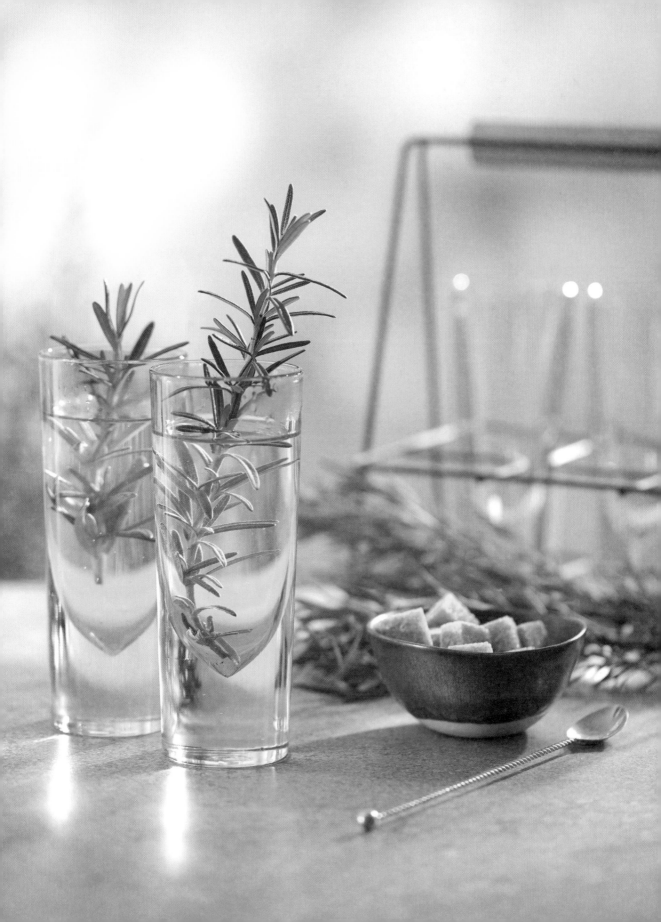

Lavender

(Lavandula angustifolia)

Wander past a lavender bush in summer and it's hard to resist breathing in a little deeper for a lungful of its soothing, perfumed aroma. Just a couple of flower heads is all it takes to export that fragrance to a mug of hot liquid, letting you re-create that relaxing summer scent wherever you are.

GROW IT

Garden centers and nurseries are stocked with a huge range of lavenders, from the frilly butterfly looks of French lavender to cultivars that come in white and pink. For culinary purposes, seek the old-fashioned purple English lavender (*Lavandula angustifolia*). Growing from seed can be slow and erratic, and larger plants are often expensive, but it's easy to propagate from cuttings. Small plants will grow quickly, reaching full size in 2–3 years.

Like most Mediterranean plants, they like sun and good drainage, so add some horticultural vermiculite to heavy soil and plant on a slight mound if you can. You can trim the soft growth after flowering to keep it in shape or let it grow wild and woody.

BREW IT

A little lavender goes a long way—just 2–3 flower heads (or 1 teaspoon of dried flowers) will be enough for a mug of hot water. Dry the flower heads still attached to their stalks—you can tie them in bunches and suspend them in a warm room—and then pick the flowers off before storing.

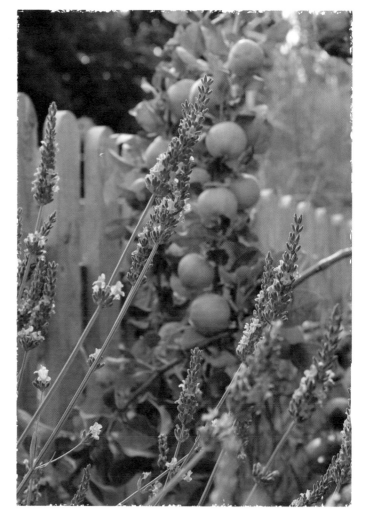

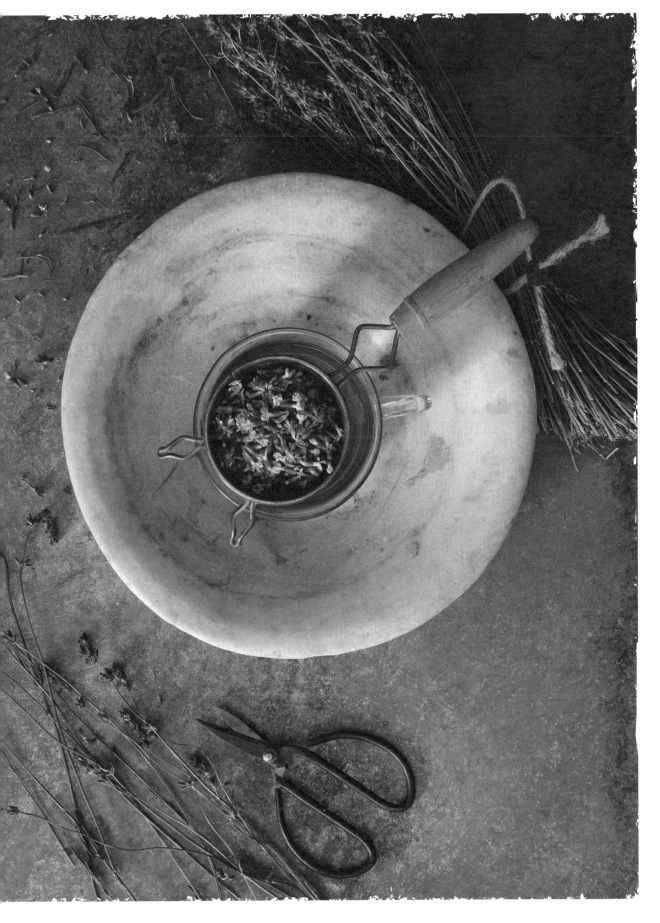

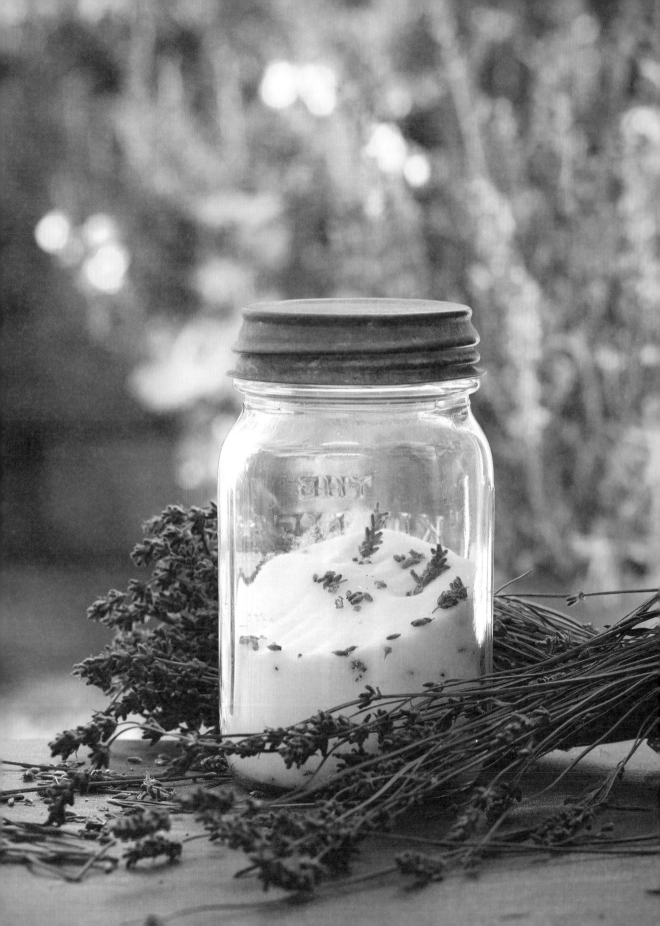

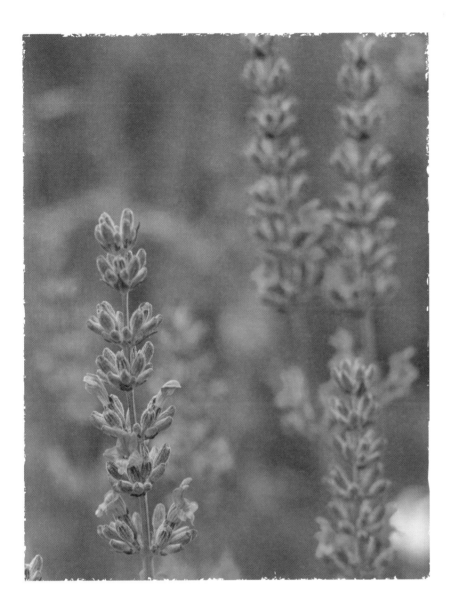

You can drink lavender tea on its own, but we find it more effective to add its aromatic charms to another hot drink. Its soothing skills are even more noticeable when working in tandem with milk, so add some to a milky black tea, chai, latte or just a mug of hot milk.

HEALTH BENEFITS

The calming fragrance of lavender has long been used by aromatherapists to help treat anxiety, and some people use it to ease a headache.

BLEND IT

Lavender is often combined with other calming herbs, such as lemon balm, and regularly features in floral blends. We like it simply infused into black tea; sprinkle a few teaspoons of flowers into an 8-ounce package of loose tea (about 3 cups) and let them work their magic for a few days before brewing.

LAVENDER SUGAR

A great way to get your lavender fix in teas (or cookies, cakes, and desserts) is to make lavender sugar. Simply mix a couple of teaspoons of lavender flowers into 1 cup of sugar and let them infuse for a few days before using.

Hyssop
(*Hyssopus officinalis*)

This herbaceous perennial is a relative of mint and has a menthol flavoring that certainly reminds us of its family friend. But it also brings its own unique characteristics, possessing an unusually spicy, bitter edge that makes it great for teas. Its shrubby, evergreen good looks are well suited to garden borders and the bees love it, too, with apiarists using it to produce an intense honey that could just be the perfect sweetener for your healthy drinks.

GROW IT

Hyssop is easy to cultivate from seed and grows quickly, eventually becoming a small shrub with woody stems. It likes well-drained soil and some sunshine, and it is rarely troubled by pests. Its spikes of flowers are commonly a purply blue, but they can also be pink, red, or white. Not to be confused with anise hyssop (see *page 114*).

BREW IT

You can make tea from hyssop's leaves and flowers, although we only use the former and save the flowers for our insect friends instead. The leaves are tiny, so you'll need a few, either fresh or dry, to fill 1 teaspoon for a cup of tea. Just fill the cup with hot water and, for some invigorating freshness, a squeeze of lemon juice.

HEALTH BENEFITS

Hyssop has something of a medicinal smell,* so it's not surprising it has been a common ingredient in various remedies for centuries. Its main use has been to stave off impending colds, while some folk also take it to clear their phlegmy passages once a cold has struck. It has been claimed to be good for (among other things) the digestive system, blood flow, as a calming aid, an immune system booster, and a treatment for cuts, sores, bites, and stings. If all this is true, then you can have an entire medicine cabinet in just one plant.

BLEND IT

Hyssop's punchy flavors and medicinal aromas make it a good alternative (or partner) to mint in healthy herbal concoctions.

DID YOU KNOW?

Hyssop is a key ingredient in several herbal liqueurs, notably Chartreuse and Bénédictine, and its aromatic charms are also used in eau de colognes.

---

* *In centuries gone by, it was used like an ancient form of bleach to clean rooms that had a whiff of sickness to them. And even farther back in time, it was used as a holy herb to purge the souls of wrongdoing.*

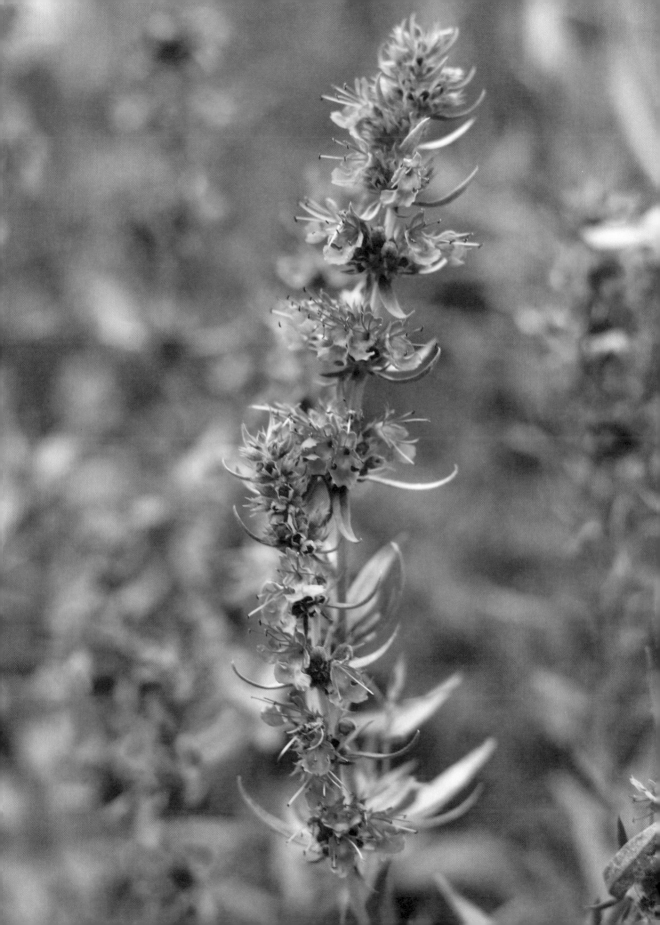

Nettle

(Urtica dioica)

Nettle can be one of the most frustrating plants for foragers. It's abundant where it grows, versatile, delicious, and nutritious, but grab a handful in passing and you'll be covered in painful stings. It's worth the effort of tackling the venomous weed with gloves and scissors—you can harvest a whole load of leaves quickly and make one of the most popular wild teas around.

FORAGE IT

Nettles love the cool, damp climate, such as in Washington State, but they are adaptable enough to attempt world domination, growing just about everywhere. They usually cover large areas, particularly on the edges of cultivated land, and the leaves are at their best when they emerge in spring.

BREW IT

The leaves' tannic astringency and green vitality make a tea that instantly tastes healthy and refreshing. Young leaves are best, so pick in early spring or use the tips (the top two sets of leaves) later in the year. Just 2–3 fresh tips, steeped in boiling water for 5 minutes, make a great cup of tea. The leaves are also excellent dried*—their flavors significantly intensify and just 1 teaspoon, steeped for 5 minutes, is enough for a tea.

HEALTH BENEFITS

Nettles are crammed with minerals and nutrients, including iron and vitamin C, making the tea a healthy and invigorating tonic. Among its apparent benefits are a treatment for hay fever (and other allergies), boosting immunity, reducing blood sugar, treating anemia, and detoxifying kidneys. If only they provided a cure for stings.

WHITE DEAD NETTLE

Nettle's stingless lookalike has bright white flowers clustered around its leaves and is also suitable for making tea. Again, it's the tips you need, and you can also include the flowers.
If you're eagerly foraging before the flowers are out, there are two ways of telling it apart from the stinging nettle:

1. Look at the stems; the dead nettle's are square and hollow, the stinging nettle's are round and solid.

2. Grab a handful.

Be careful when drying your own, for even a crispy dry nettle leaf can sting.

BLEND IT

Those tannins in the dried leaves are excellent for a wide variety of teas and go with most other ingredients. You'll commonly find them in healthy herbal blends.

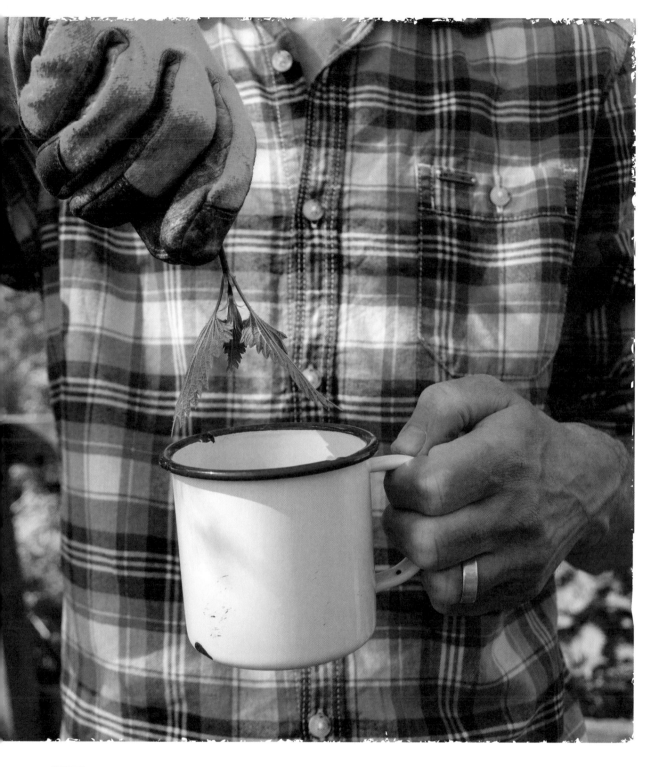

DID YOU KNOW?

The nettle's sting is caused by a combination of neurotransmitters and acids at the tips of its hairy leaves. Some nettle-related oddness occurs every year in Dorset, England, where a pub holds the World Nettle Eating Championships in which competitors see who can eat the most leaves.

Lemon Verbena

(Aloysia citrodora)

This large, deciduous shrub of South America is arguably the king of lemon-scented plants (actual lemon trees aside). Lemon verbena's strong lemon smell is due to the essential oils that reside in its leaves. Try rubbing a fresh leaf between your finger and thumb and give it a good sniff—it's like sticking your nose in a big bag of lemon boiled candies, an aroma that transfers magnificently well to wild tea.

GROW IT

Lemon verbena is a tender plant more suited to hot areas. In warm areas, if yours are in the ground, mulch and protect them from frosts. Move container plants indoors from fall. If your plant appears skeletal and lifeless after winter, hold back from hurling it toward the compost pile, because new growth takes time to appear and it may well rise like Lazarus in late spring.

BREW IT

Use 3–4 freshly picked leaves per cup of boiled water, bruising them first before dropping them in. Essential oils held in the leaves help this herb to retain its zingy lemon taste, which becomes even stronger after air drying—try using 1–2 teaspoons of dried leaves per cup.

HEALTH BENEFITS

Lemon verbena has long been used as a mild sedative; its high antioxidant properties have been known to reduce muscle damage during exercise. Try filling your water bottle with cold lemon verbena tea for your morning run—it might help ease your achy legs and joints.

BLEND IT

Fresh leaves add a citrusy punch to iced teas, while the dried leaves are excellent for injecting lemon flavor into blends in place of actual lemons.

MORE LEMONY PLANTS TO TRY

Lemon Balm (*Melissa officinalis*)
A large-leafed lemon-scented herb, perfect for tea-making purposes (see *opposite*).

Lemongrass (*Cymbopogon citratus*)
Its edible stems are widely used in Asian cuisine, and the leaves make a great tea (see *page 108*). It likes hot climes and hates frosts.

Lemon Basil (*Ocimum × citriodorum*)
A hybrid of American basil and sweet basil. Infuse it in olive oil for a flavorsome dipping oil for crusty bread. Nick declares this variety his favorite basil for tea making.

Lemon Balm

(Melissa officinalis)

This bushy, rampant perennial belongs to the mint family. You'll often spy it lurking in kitchen plots, where it is grown to lend lemony flavors to savory dishes, salads, and sauces. As well as boasting excellent culinary credentials, lemon balm has enjoyed a long association with beekeepers. Bees can't get enough of this zesty plant, so it has historically been placed near beehives to placate the apian inhabitants and to hopefully prevent them from swarming off to new pastures. The clue is in the name: *Melissa officinalis* stems from the Greek word *melissa*, meaning "honeybee."

GROW IT

Lemon balm loves most soil types and will grow in shade or full sun. It's an invasive plant, so keep it in check by cutting back the plant after it flowers. This will also encourage fresh growth, which makes the best tea. If things get really out of hand and it starts to swamp surrounding plants, lift and divide clumps in fall.

BREW IT

The leaves of lemon balm tend to lose their aroma when dried, so if you have easy access to a plant, use them fresh, harvesting just before the plant starts to bear flowers for maximum fragrance. Try infusing 2 teaspoons of leaves in a mug full of freshly boiled water for 5–10 minutes.

HEALTH BENEFITS

Lemon balm contains eugenol, an aromatic, oily liquid that has both anesthetic and antiseptic qualities. You may find it stuffed into hop pillows, along with lavender, chamomile, and the obligatory hop to aid and improve sleep for people who experience insomnia.

BLEND IT

Try mixing fresh lemon balm leaves with some of its minty pals. Our preferred pairing is with peppermint, where it brings a fresh citric zip to proceedings. Folk with a sweet tooth should add a spoonful of honey in homage to this bee-loved balm.

DID YOU KNOW?

Not all insects are as enamored with lemon balm as bees. Mosquitoes positively hate it, so gardeners who are regularly pestered by these biting bugs should rub a crushed handful of leaves over exposed skin to keep them at bay.

Chamomile

(Matricaria recutita)

Chamomile is an herbal tea trailblazer that has been available in grocery and health food stores long before most other wild brews got in on the act. If you want to grow your own, there are two types you'll probably encounter, German chamomile (*Matricaria recutita*) and Roman chamomile (*Chamaemelum nobile*). Roman chamomile is the low-lying, ragged-looking one (also known as the ground apple) and the one you need to choose if you want to plant a fragrant (yet maintenance heavy) chamomile lawn. It's the German species that we've had the most success with in our community garden. It also happens to be the one most widely used for medicinal purposes and, more important, the best for making tasty tea.

FORAGE IT

German chamomile is native to southern and eastern Europe and western Asia. However, German chamomile has been introduced to several states spread across the country, so there is a chance that you could find it on your foraging excursions, or to a lesser extent, you just might stumble across Roman chamomile, which grows in the wild in a few states.

GROW IT

Chamomile will grow well from seed, which is best started in trays, with the young seedlings transplanted into the ground when big enough to handle. Both Roman and German chamomile are adaptable to most growing conditions, but German chamomile tends to be a little more rugged and will grow in poor soil conditions. Unlike its ground hugging Roman cousin, German chamomile stands upright and can reach heights of more than 2 feet. Clip your plants regularly during the growing season to prevent them from becoming leggy, and keep them well watered to prevent them from drying out.

BREW IT

You can use either fresh or dried flowers, but using fresh ones will give you a fruitier brew, plus you'll get an instant fix without having spent the time drying them. Don't overdo it, because too many flowers will make a bitter beverage. Try using 3–4 flower heads in a cup of hot water for starters and see how you get on. Let them infuse for 5 minutes, strain, then sip.

DID YOU KNOW?

Chamomile tea can be used as a face wash to help treat acne. Just use the recipe for brewing (see left), remembering to FIRST LET IT COOL.

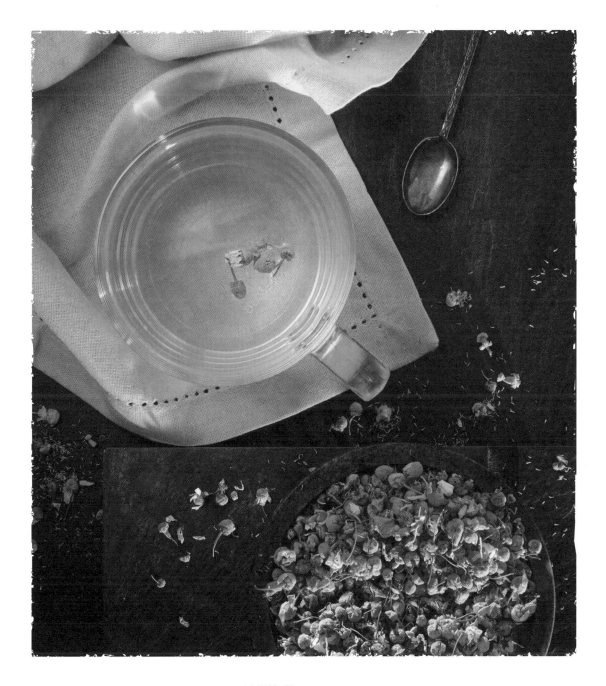

HEALTH BENEFITS

Chamomile tea is highly prized for its
reported calming properties. Some folk
also take it to relax their muscles and
to ease aches and pains, making it a
favorite beverage for gardeners to drink
after a hard day's work.

BLEND IT

Try blending chamomile as part of a
floral blend. Lavender works well, as
does a rose petal/green tea combo.
Adding lemon balm helps bring out
the fruity flavors—and it smells
incredible, too.

Bee Balm

(*Monarda didyma*)

Bee balm is one of the many names given to monarda, a striking herbaceous plant that possesses bee-alluring pollen. Another of its aliases is bergamot, because its leaves possess an aroma similar to the bergamot fruit. It's this latter quality that earns it a place in our top 40 and, although you can also use the flowers for tea, we prefer to leave them to the bees and plunder the greenery instead.

GROW IT

There are annual bee balm plants out there, but we're devoting our attention to the perennial *Monarda didyma*. Although it shouldn't be too difficult to grow, we've found it to be one of those fussy plants that will decide it doesn't want to bother for seemingly no reason. It likes to be kept watered in good, well-drained soil, but will throw a tantrum if it dries out (in summer) or sits in excessive water (especially over winter). It likes a little space to grow, but after a few years, it will spread to the point where it needs to be dug up and split into smaller plants. Deadhead flowers in summer to extend the blooming season, then cut the plant to the ground in fall. A spring mulch will get it up and running again.

BREW IT

Bee balm's leaves have an unusual aromatic orange fragrance, similar to the bergamot fruit, along with some herby qualities, with thyme most often coming to mind. We think its aromas and flavors are enhanced by drying the leaves, but you can also use them fresh. Either way, 1–2 teaspoons of chopped leaves added to a cup of boiling water and steeped for at least 5 minutes makes a good tea.

BLEND IT

Those bergamot similarities see it used as an alternative to the fruit's oil in an approximation of Earl Grey (see *page 125*) and you can also mix it with lemon and orange peel to enhance those citrusy characteristics.

HEALTH BENEFITS

Monarda didyma hails from North America and has been a traditional remedy for skin and mouth-related ailments among Native Americans, because the plant contains thymol, an ingredient that regularly features in mouthwashes. It has also been used by some folk in their own personal battles with flatulence.

TOP TIP

Bee balm benefits from a "Chelsea chop"—the hacking back of some plants post-Chelsea Flower Show (a popular flower show in London that takes place in late May) to encourage more vigorous growth. Lop off the top two-thirds of your bee balm plants, and turn the leaves into a stockpile of dried tea.

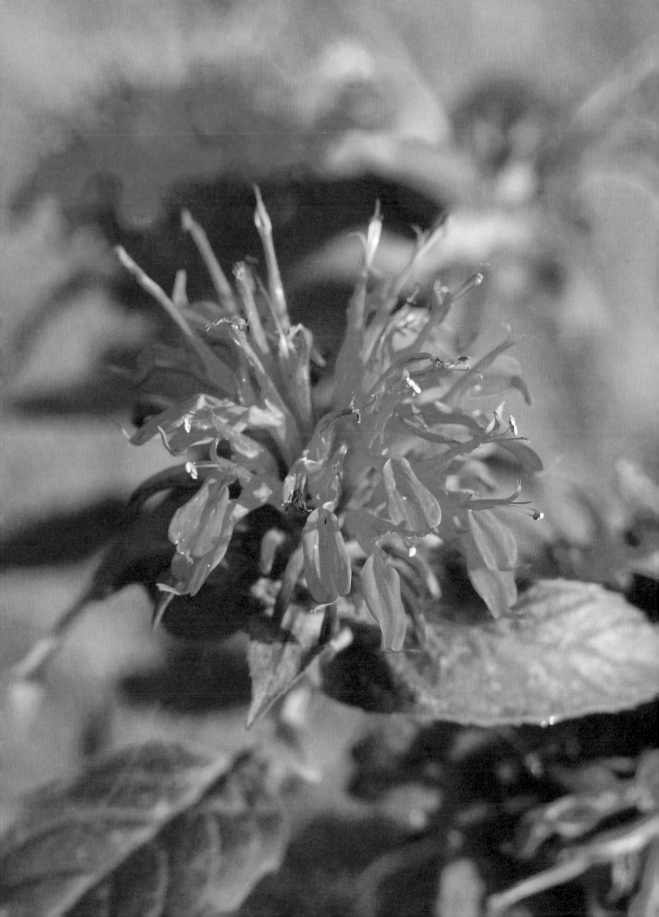

Pot Marigold

(Calendula officinalis)

Pot marigold seems to have fallen out of gardening fashion, frequently overlooked in favor of showier cultivars of French and African marigolds (from the *Tagetes* genus). But these fancier flowers lack one key feature for us—they're not edible. It's the simpler sunshine colors of the pot marigold that brightens up our garden and adds a splash of color to our teas.

GROW IT

There are loads of *Calendula officinalis* cultivars available in a full range of sunny colors, from vibrant yellows to deep oranges (and with a few pale peachy pinks for good measure), but it's worth tracking down the original pot marigold, which has a vivid mid-orange hue. Sowing this annual from its squiggly-looking seed is easy (a successful crop will probably self-seed the following year), and a healthy plant should flower from early summer through to the first frosts. It looks good in both containers and borders.

BREW IT

You can make tea with the leaves and green parts of the flowers, but they can be an irritant to the throat, so it's best to use the petals. If you're drying them, pick the whole flowers and pluck the petals when they've completely dried out. On their own, the petals make a delicious but delicate brew, so infuse 1–2 teaspoons (fresh or dried) for at least 5 minutes in a cup of hot water. It could be a psychological thing, but we think the yellow strands not only look like saffron but taste a little like it, too, with a slightly sweet and earthy flavor.

HEALTH BENEFITS

Pot marigold has antibacterial properties and has traditionally been used to treat skin ailments, such as burns, bites, stings, and itchy irritations, but we don't advise pouring a mug of hot tea over any such sores. Instead, drinking it is said to provide healthy nourishment to your skin and is used to help ease a sore throat.

BLEND IT

Those delicate flavors make it hard for pot marigold to shine in any tea blends, although it does often appear in floral brews, especially those devised for their health benefits.

DID YOU KNOW?

Marigold petals have long been used in cooking as a colorful saffron substitute and to provide a yellow tinge to foodstuffs, such as cheese and butter. They are also used to thicken and flavor pots of soup and stews—it's for this reason the plant got its "pot" marigold name.

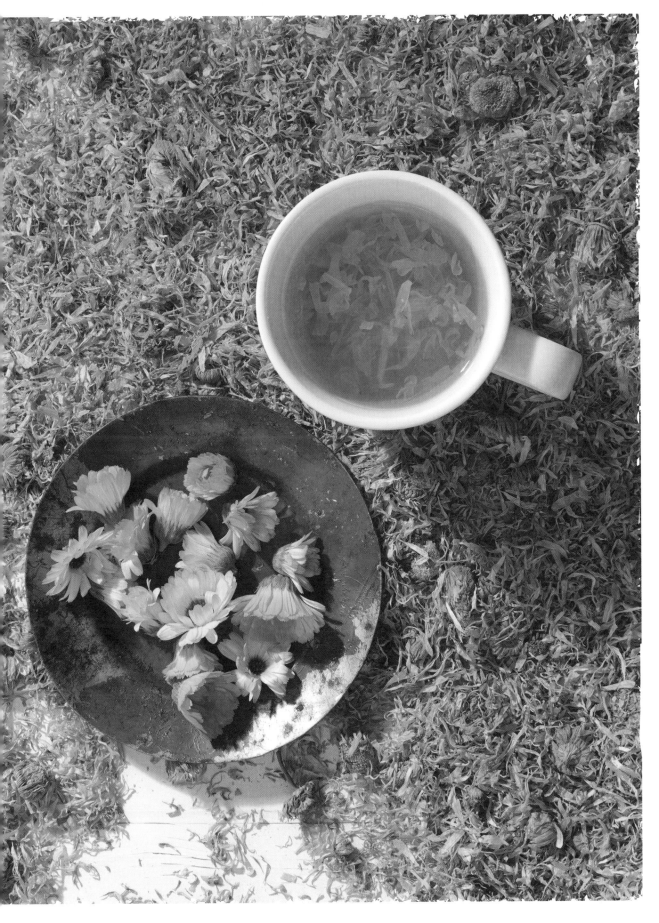

Sweet Fennel

(Foeniculum vulgare)

If you like the taste of anise, then grow some fennel. Every part of this magnificent plant—leaves, flowers, seeds, stems, and roots—is infused with its flavor, and hot water is all you need to add for a mug of aniselike goodness. But the perennial herb is not only packed with flavor, it also has great visual appeal, with a vast web of lush green fronds in spring, followed by masses of yellow flowers in summer.

GROW IT

Fennel is a member of the carrot family, and there are two edible types you can grow.* Florence fennel is cultivated for its bulbs, which swell while growing, although we've found it a difficult plant on our patch and rarely get much girth before it bolts. Instead, we grow the much larger and more spectacular sweet fennel, also known as herb fennel, wild fennel, or common fennel.

It's best sown in situ early in the year and is easy to grow (although given the choice, it will opt for sunshine and well-drained soil). Plants can reach up to 10 feet tall, so it will hog a large corner of your yard, but it's such a handsome-looking plant that it's well worth giving up the space.

FORAGE IT

Due to its bullying size and the ease at which it self-seeds, fennel is often seen as an unwanted invader when it appears in the wild. If you're out on a fennel foraging mission. then your best bet is to hunt around recently broken areas of ground, alongside roads, or sites close to the coast.

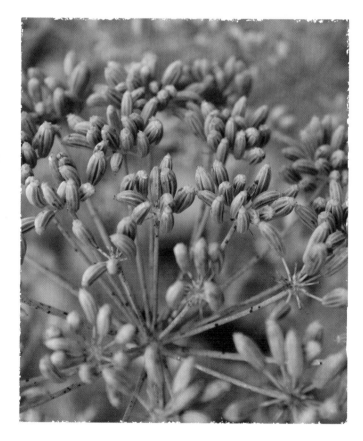

* A similar plant, giant fennel (Ferula communis), can be poisonous, and another carrot relative, Crithmum maritimum, is known as sea fennel.

BREW IT

You could try digging up the roots to brew with, but it's a lot of effort for minimum rewards when there's a vast plant on top that comes back year after year to give you plenty of tea-making opportunities. The seeds are the highlight, with 1 teaspoon surrendering plenty of flavor when infused in a mug of hot water for at least 5 minutes (lightly crack them first with a mortar and pestle for maximum effect). Before the seeds are ready, you can steep the frilly leaves in a cup of hot water for 5–10 minutes—simply grab a small handful (stems included) and coarsely chop before infusing.

HEALTH BENEFITS

Fennel is most commonly used as a digestive aid and appears in numerous concoctions promoting women's health, with attention given to its supposed abilities to ease period pains. It's also found in teas designed for new mothers, because it is said to help increase their production of breast milk (see *page 129*).

BLEND IT

Fennel seeds are a versatile ingredient for the wild tea maker, working particularly well in spicy drinks (see our chai recipes on *page 130*), or for adding some sweet anise flavors to herbal brews.

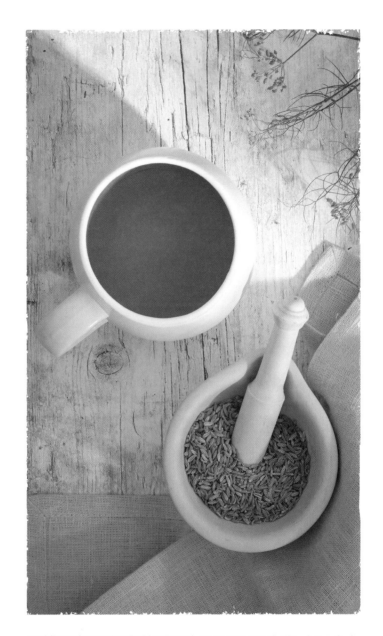

WHEN TO HARVEST SEEDS

In late fall, the fennel seeds (technically the plant's fruit) will begin to ripen. The best time to pick them is when their green color has faded and begins to show light shades of brown (if you leave them too long, they'll get browner and start to fall off or turn soggy from rain). Pick the whole flower head, rub the seeds into a bowl, and remove any parts of stalky debris (and bugs) before storing in an airtight container.

Echinacea

(Echinacea angustifolia, E. purpurea)

Echinacea is an herbaceous plant that has been used as a medicinal tea by Native Americans for centuries. *Echniacea purpurea* is more commonly known as purple coneflower, although not all culitvars are purple. Its large blooms sit on tall, sturdy stems, which has made it as popular in flower borders as in the medicine cabinet. Grow it yourself and you'll have to wrestle with the conundrum of whether to enjoy its visual delights or chop it up and drink it instead.

GROW IT

There are many echinacea cultivars and hybrids, but tea makers should choose the two most often used in medicine: *Echinacea angustifolia* and *E. purpurea*. They like conditions akin to those found in the prairies—hot and bare—where they grow wild, so give them your sunniest spot and try not to overcrowd them with other plants. They will need plenty of room below ground for their deep roots to burrow, making them less effective in containers. To increase your stock, you can divide established plants in spring or fall.

BREW IT

It's echinacea's roots that are most commonly used, but you can also make teas from the leaves, flowers, and seeds. It seems a shame to dig up plants to harvest the roots, especially because cleaning and preparing them is tricky, so we use the leaves. Steep 1 teaspoon of leaves in a cup of boiling water for 5 minutes to make the tea. The most noticeable property of echinacea tea is the tingling sensation it gives your tongue. We think it's more suited to blends than drinking on its own.

HEALTH BENEFITS

Echinacea has been a superherb for Native Americans, who traditionally use it to treat a myriad of ailments, from sore throats and toothache to scorpion stings and snakebites. These days it has become a general well-being remedy that's used in all kinds of flu and cold potions.

BLEND IT

It works well with other floral teas (it will benefit from their aroma, while they'll appreciate echinacea's earthy and tongue-tingling properties) and with other cold-fighting ingredients, such as rose hips and elderberries, which come packed with vitamin C (see *page 129*).

DID YOU KNOW?

The genus name *Echinacea* is derived from the Greek word for "hedgehog," (*ekhinos*) because the flower's center looks like the spiny mammal.

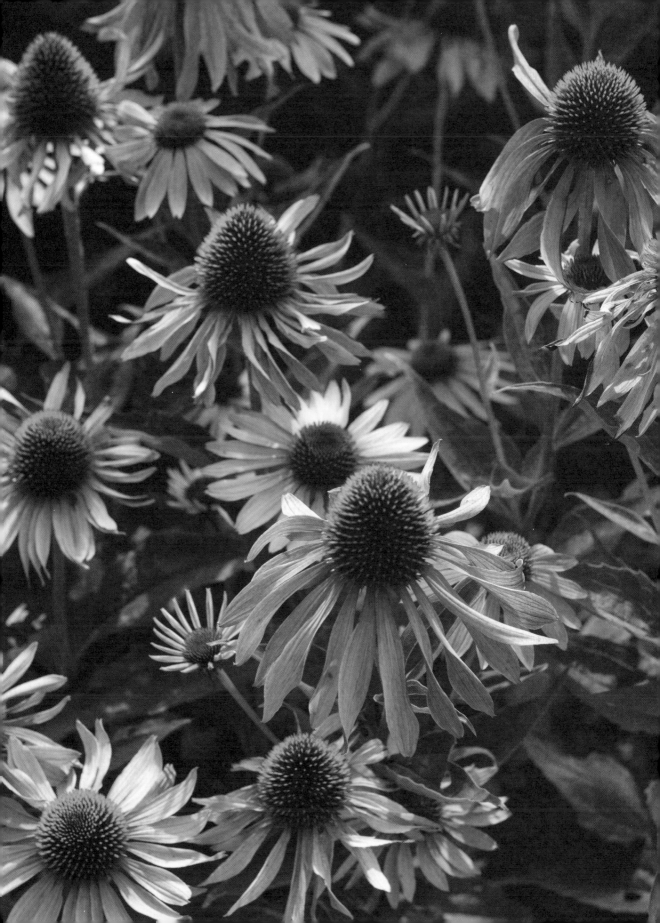

Corn

(Zea mays)

Corn is one of the best vegetables to grow yourself. Few things taste as good as a ripe ear of corn freshly snapped from its stalk and plunged straight into boiling water or put onto a barbecue grill. If only there was something you could do with the ear's flowing mane of corn silks. Well actually there is.

GROW IT

Corn is a reliable grower from seed and, providing your plants get ample sun and water, you should have little trouble from them. Corn uses the wind to pollinate, so it needs to be planted in blocks—if you grow it in a row and the wind blows in the wrong direction, your ears will be cornless. You also have to keep an eye open for mammals stealing the goods—those golden ears are particularly attractive to deer and raccoons, and rodents can strip the sweet niblets from an ear in practically no time.

BREW IT

A tea made from roasted corn is popular in Korea. It involves cooking the kernels in boiling water for just a few minutes, then thoroughly drying them before slowly roasting until they are almost black. These are then ground and used as a tea. It's so popular in Korea that you can readily buy roasted corn tea bags.

For a much simpler brew, you can also use the corn silks—the hairy tassels that flow from each ear.* You can wrench the corn silks from the cobs once the kernels have started to turn golden yellow and use them fresh or dried. Simply trim away any brown or ratty looking ends and put 1 tablespoon of fresh silks (when scrunched up) or 2 teaspoons of dried silks in a mug and cover with boiling water for 2–3 minutes. The tea has a sweet and mild cornlike flavor that you may want to pep up with a sliver of ginger.

HEALTH BENEFITS

Corn silks have been used as a traditional medicine for centuries, due to the belief that they have diuretic properties that can flush the system of toxins and help with urinary and kidney problems (although there doesn't seem to be a whole lot of substantiated research available to back this up).

BLEND IT

We think corn silk is best used as a background flavor for brews with spices, such as ginger, or it can be blended with Roasted Barley Tea (see page 144) to add some sweetness to the more bitter barley.

* The Latin name for corn silks is Stigmata maydis, which means "mother's hair." This, and "ear hair," don't sound as appetizing to us as "corn silks."

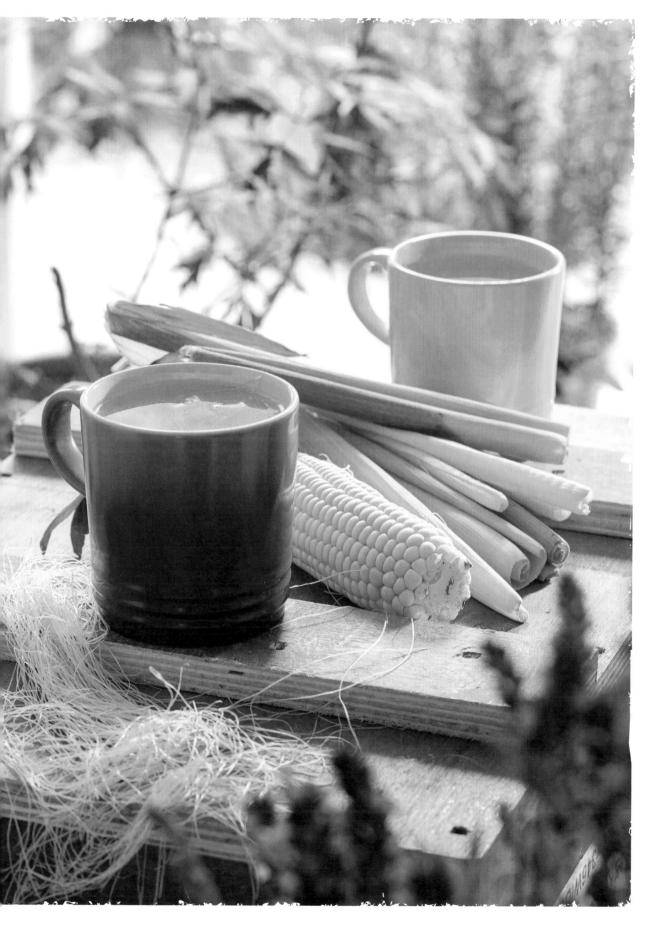

Oats

(*Avena sativa*)

Oats are an odd choice to have growing in a community garden. They are usually sprouting in vast fields on an industrial scale, destined to be pummeled into porridge, or made into animal fodder to feed hungry ruminants. Down on the plot, we've surrendered a raised bed for their cultivation. They make a fine sight, swaying in the breeze under the soft, golden glow of a late summer sun, but our real interest lies in beverages. Our oats are grown for beer-making experiments and to provide us with the necessary ingredients for a tasty, wholesome cup of tea.

GROW IT

Oats are an annual plant and can be sown in hot regions in fall (for a late summer harvest) or in cold regions in spring (for an early fall harvest). Sow the seed in shallow rows, or use the tried and trusted, old-school method of scattering them randomly with a flick of the wrist. Lightly cover the area with soil or run the risk of birds hoovering up the seed before they germinate. Oats grow vigorously and densely, so you shouldn't have many problems with weeds once established.

When growing for maximum yield, farmers harvest the oat grains just after the last green kernels start to turn cream. Overripe grains tend to detach easily from the plant and you'll lose a lot to the soil when gathering mechanically on an industrial scale. For tea-making purposes, you'll need the whole plant (except the roots), so you don't need to be so precise with timings. Wait until the grains turn golden and harvest using a sharp knife, cutting the plant about an inch above soil level.

BREW IT

Oats need some coaxing to release their goodness. Chop up a couple of handfuls of oats (leaves, stems, and kernels), pour over boiling water, and steep overnight. In the morning, reheat your oaty brew in a saucepan, then pour it through a strainer into a cup. Oat kernels alone can be used to make a tasty milk alternative (see *page 24*)

HEALTH BENEFITS

One of the major benefits of eating oats is that they lower cholesterol, thanks to the soluble fiber they contain. Oat straw tea is also believed to be a brain booster that can improve mental performance. They are also full of melatonin, which can make you sleepy—just ask Goldilocks.

BLEND IT

We think oats work well with lemony additions, so try them with lemon verbena or lemon balm. Oat straw and mint also make an interesting combination.

DID YOU KNOW?

Oats are the staple grain of Scotland, because unlike fussy old wheat, they thrive in the country's cold, wet, and humid climate.

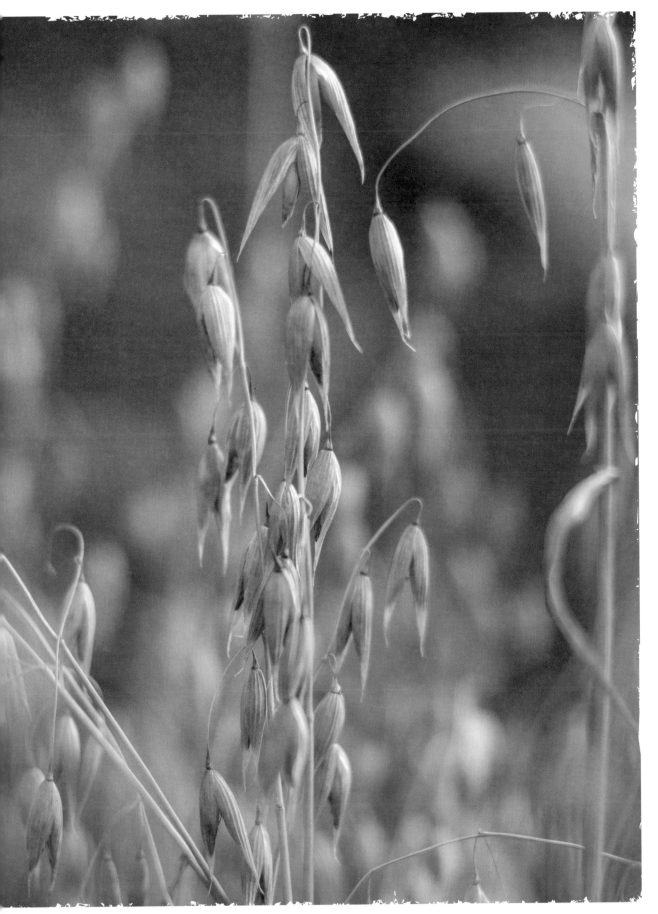

Rose

(*Rosa*)

With edible flowers and fruit, a rosebush can provide rich pickings for the thirsty gardener. As a general rule, petals plucked from the more fragrant cultivars are often the best for turning into tea. An obvious and aptly named candidate for the pot is the tea rose, because its spicy fragrance is similar to that of black tea. We also make fine floral brews from the fruit, with the dog rose (*Rosa canina*) being one of our favorites. We once regarded it as an unwelcome community-garden guest, because of its tendency to entangle our precious hop bines. We now spare it from a savage trim with shears and welcome our new brewing buddy with open arms.

FORAGE IT

Depending on where you live, the dog rose is one of the species you may come across when out foraging. It's also known as the wild rose, and it'll be furious when you start picking its petals. Don't bag them all for yourself; leave a few flower heads on the plant for insects to enjoy. Make a mental note of the location of the plants you discover, because you may want to return later in the year to gather rose hips for more brewing action or to make rose hip syrup for bubble tea (see *page 166*).

GROW IT

Roses are a hardy breed and will thrive in most soil conditions. They like plenty of sunshine and are not too great on windy sites. They can be thirsty fellas, so keep them well watered to promote healthy growth and to prolong the flowering period. Deadheading your roses is an essential (and satisfying)

part of healthy plant management. Go around your bush after the flowers have finished blooming and snip off any dead heads with a sharp pair of secateurs; you can cut back each flowering stem as far as three sets of leaves. Hip-sters who are looking forward to foraging rose hips should skip the deadheading and allow the fruit to form in peace.

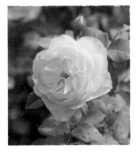

BREW THE PETALS

A tea made solely from rose petals smells great but is subtle on the palate, so it's best to blend them with green or black tea leaves to bring out those floral flavors (see Tea Twists, *page 125*).

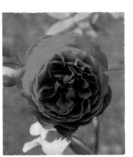

BREW THE HIPS

Rose hips are the real star of the show and pack stacks of vitamin C, making them the perfect fruity addition to a healthy brew (see *page 128*). Coarsely

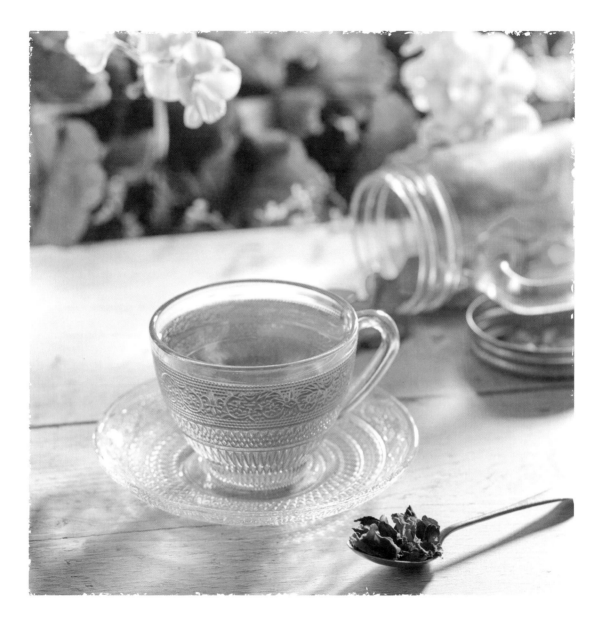

chop and dry the fruit, add 1 teaspoon to a cup, and fill with hot water, then let infuse for 5–10 minutes. Make sure you strain the tea thoroughly before serving, because the tiny hairs found inside rose hips can irritate the throat.

HEALTH BENEFITS

The health-giving properties of the rose are not to be sniffed at. Rose tea is high in vitamin C, which can stimulate the production of the white blood cells that play a key role in fighting infections.

BLEND IT

Hawthorn leaves and wild rose petals make a refreshing, lightly floral brew; try a 3 to 1 mix (in favor of the rose petal). Dried and ground rose hips can add fruity flavors to any number of healthy tonics.

Ginger

(Zingiber officinale)

Ginger is an indispensable ingredient for the aspiring drinks maker. A native of Southeast Asia, the plant in the wild produces elegant, conelike flowers. The part we are concerned with, however, is the root— the technically inaccurate name given to the knobbly, hand-shape rhizome from which the plant's stems sprout.

GROW IT

Growing ginger is a protracted affair—to be honest, you are probably better off foraging it from your local grocery store. It can be done, however, if you are prepared to be patient. Go to the store and select a piece of ginger, ideally one that already has small green buds forming. Wash it, cut off the part with the bud, and put it into a tall plant pot filled with some horticultural vermiculite added to a potting mix on a sunny windowsill. Green shoots should start to appear in a few weeks, and after 6–8 months you should notice a bulbous swelling where the shoots meet the soil. This is the rhizome, and the part which we crave. Eventually the foliage of your plants will die down and you can harvest the root, although you may want to let the plant develop larger rhizomes and pick them the following year. Dry the root somewhere dark and cool until its outer skin turns papery, but remember to save some to continue the growing cycle.

BREW IT

Add ½ cup of freshly grated ginger root to a cup, add boiling water to fill the cup, and let steep for 10 minutes. Strain before serving, adding a slice of lemon and honey to taste.

HEALTH BENEFITS

Ginger has long been used as a treatment for an upset stomach and many people take it as a cure for travel sickness. It also contains powerful anti-inflammatory compounds called gingerols, which can help soothe sore muscles and joints.

BLEND IT

Ginger has a tendency to boss whatever it is paired with, so use it sparingly or fight fire with fire and combine it with a pinch or two of chili powder for a real zinger of a brew. It's a common feature of winter-warming brews and spicy chais (see *page 130*) and works well with ingredients with a sharp flavor, such as lemon and rhubarb (see *page 167*). It's also handy for taming the taste of some of the more challenging brews, such as Bladder Wrack Tea (see *page 94*).

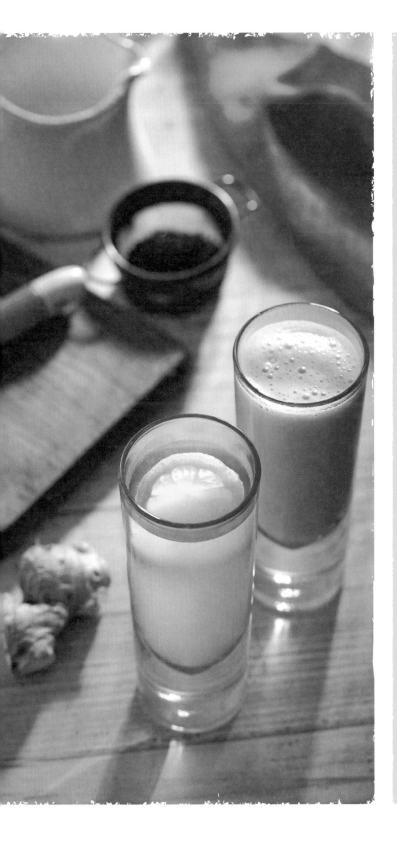

GINGER TEAS

Sliced, grated, or peeled? Everyone has a favorite way of making ginger tea. Here are three recipes to try:

TEH HALIA
Malaysia

1 Peel and bruise a 1-inch piece of ginger.
2 Boil 1 cup of water in a small saucepan, add the ginger, and simmer for 10 minutes.
3 Remove the ginger from the pan, remove the pan from the heat, and add 1 teaspoon of black tea.
4 Let brew for 5 minutes, strain, then add a splash of condensed milk to serve.

SAENGGANG-CHA
Korea

1 Peel and thinly slice a 1-inch piece of ginger.
2 Boil 1 cup of water in a small saucepan, add the sliced ginger, half a cinnamon stick, and simmer for 20 minutes.
3 Strain into a cup, sweeten with honey, and serve with pine nuts.

ADRAK KI CHAI
India

1 Peel and finely grate a 1-inch piece of ginger.
2 Mix ½ cup of milk with ½ cup of water in a saucepan and bring to a boil.
3 Add the grated ginger and simmer for 5 minutes.
4 Add 1 teaspoon strong black tea, turn off the heat, and brew for 5 minutes.
5 Serve with honey to taste.

Lemon

(Citrus limon)

The sharp, acidic bite of lemon can cut through all flavors, lending its zesty refreshment to a number of hot and cold drinks. With its versatility ranging from classic lemon tea to a soothing honey and lemon mix or invigorating lemon and ginger, everyone should make sure they always have a lemon or two on hand.

GROW IT

Lemons like to grow in sun and warmth throughout the year, but even if you don't live in Florida or California, it's possible to grow a lemon tree in a container outdoors in summer and bring it into a heated sunroom or greenhouse in the winter. If you lack such a facility, simply rely on store-bought lemons., but wash off any wax coatings in warm water before use.

BREW IT

There are many ways to add a burst of zesty lemon freshness to drinks: a squirt of juice straight into a cup, a slice as a flavorsome garnish, or adding dried zest to a blend (see box, right, for ideas). For the simplest, purest lemon tea, simply steep 2 slices in a cup of hot water for 5 minutes and serve hot or ice cold.

HEALTH BENEFITS

Lemon's most well-known health benefit is its abundance of antioxidants, notably vitamin C, which are more concentrated in the zest and pith. Start drinking it if cold bugs are circulating in your vicinity and it might just help to prevent them from striking.

BLEND IT

There aren't many ingredients that kick up a fuss when asked to share a mug with lemon. Besides the classics listed in our box, below, its acidity is also useful for adding character to simple floral teas, such as elderflower, or bringing out even more flavor from fruity brews.

FIVE WAYS WITH LEMON

The classic: Squeeze 1-2 teaspoons of fresh lemon juice into a cup of black tea (refrigerate for an iced tea).

The soother: Combine 2 teaspoons of lemon juice with 2 teaspoons of honey in a cup, then fill with hot water.

The invigorator: Chop a thumb-tip size piece of ginger and drop into a cup of hot water with a few slices of lemon.

The refresher: Add a couple of slices of lemon to a mug of mint tea.

The pick-me-up: The Portuguese drink *mazagran* is made by squeezing the juice from ½ a lemon into a cup of black coffee and sweetening it with 2 teaspoons of sugar. Best served chilled with ice.

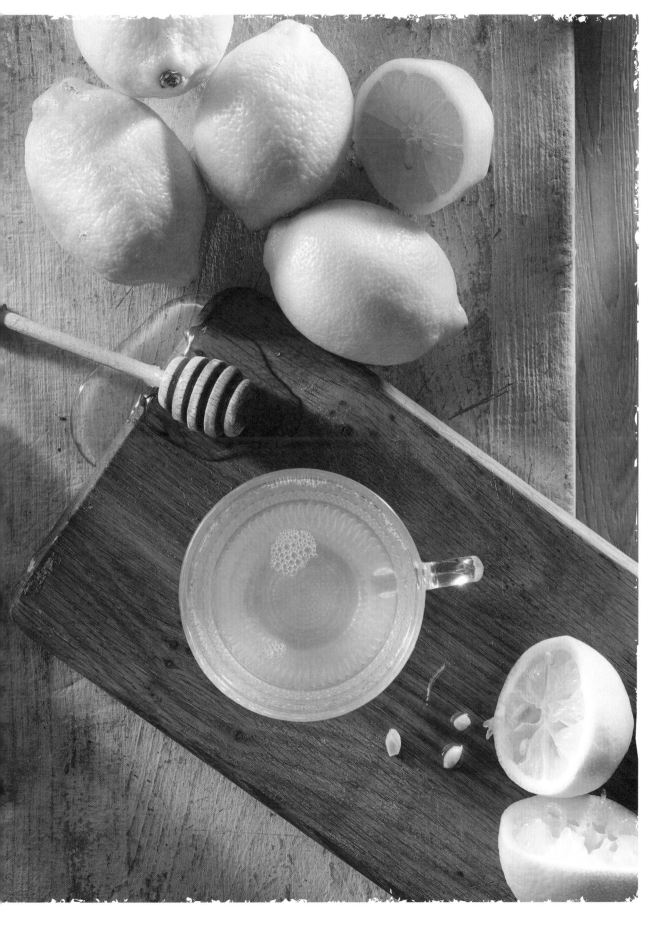

Strawberries

(Fragaria)

Speak to anyone who grows their own, and you will be told that no store-bought vegetable or fruit will ever compare to the taste of freshly grown and picked produce. While this may not be the case for all homegrown foodstuffs, there's nothing like the taste of homegrown strawberries. They are the very essence of summertime distilled into a red, fruity package. They also happen to make pretty tasty teas.

FORAGE IT

Unless you inadvertently wander through a fruit farm while out foraging, you probably won't come across the cultivated strawberries found on grocery-store shelves (for growing tips on these, see below). What you may find, however, is the wild, woodland strawberry (*Fragaria vesca*, pictured below), a small, ground-hugging plant that produces equally diminutive fruit.

Don't be fooled by their size—these strawberries have an intense, punchy flavor and the leaves of the woodland plant are the ones most often used in alternative medicine.

GROW IT

You can grow strawberry plants from seed, but the best (and easiest) option is to buy small plants. Plant them outside in early spring, preferably in

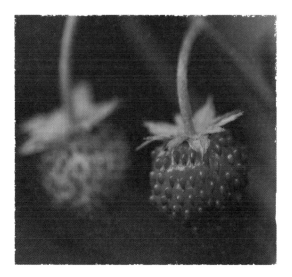

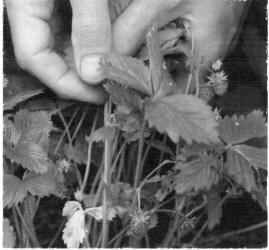

well-drained soil in a sunny position. During the summer months, just before your strawberry plants start to bear fruit, it's always good practice to lay down a bed of straw under the plants to help protect the developing fruits from slugs and other critters fond of juicy red snacks. Remove this bedding in late summer to let the plants breathe and reduce the chance of disease, then cut back your strawberry plants to 2 inches above the ground. Your plants will benefit from a generous helping of fertilizer to help them settle down for winter.

BREW IT

Strawberries are perfect for sun teas and also for syrups, which can be used to make a sweet and juicy iced tea. For an instant, delicately fragranced, pale pink cup of tea, slice 3–4 ripe strawberries (or use a small handful of whole woodland strawberries) and steep them in a cup of boiling water. They'll surrender their flavor after just a couple of minutes, and you can also invite a few strawberry leaves or some green tea to the party for extra flavor. Strain and serve hot or cold.

HEALTH BENEFITS

Colorful fruits, such as the strawberry, contain anthocyanins that are believed to have a healthy effect on the heart. Strawberries also contain decent amounts of fiber, potassium, and calcium, and their antioxidants may help support the immune system.

BLEND IT

Try adding a touch of vanilla when making a Strawberry Iced Tea (see *page* 154) for a tasty approximation of strawberries and ice cream.

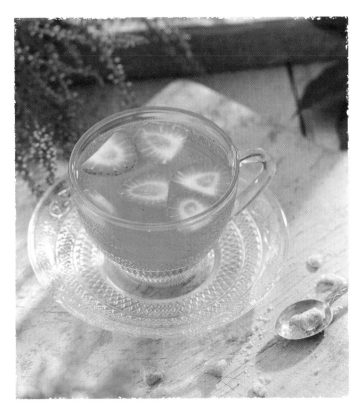

STRAWBERRY YIELDS FOREVER

A continuous supply of strawberry plants can be cultivated from a single specimen by propagating the runners (or stolons). Here's how to do it:

1. Select 2–3 runners closest to the "mother" plant and pin them down with a tent peg. Weighing them down with a small stone should also work.

2. Once the runners have taken root, which should take 4–6 weeks, carefully cut the stem from the mother plant and your new plants should begin to thrive on their own.

3. Use this technique to cultivate your strawberry beds in situ, or train individual runners into plant pots to then transport and plant elsewhere.

Apple
(*Malus*)

We live in apple country in the UK, surrounded by ancient orchards and a landscape peppered with wild trees that have grown from discarded cores. Between us, we grow eight cultivars of dessert, culinary, and cider apples, which we use for pies, alcohol, and juice, while also taking advantage of their sweet nature in a range of tasty teas.

GROW IT

If you have room in your yard for a tree, make it one of the hundreds of apple cultivars. Aim for a cultivar suited to your region and plant during the winter months while it's dormant. The first few years will be fruitless—it's best to snip off the flowers to concentrate growth in the actual tree—and the tree will need careful pruning according to the cultivar, but when established, apples need little attention.

FORAGE IT

If, like us, you're lucky enough to have apple trees growing wild near you, then keep your fingers crossed they're tasty; some are so packed with tannin they'll suck all the moisture from your cheeks, resulting in the most distorted expression you've ever had. To check if they're ripe, shake an apple and you should hear the seeds rattling; then cut one in half to see if they are brown.

BREW IT

Apples are packed with sugar and, when dried, make a rewardingly sweet and fruity addition to many blends. Apple tea is popular in Turkey and is sold simply as dried apple pieces or powdered with black tea as an "instant" drink, and it often comes flavored with spices. For your own apple tea infusion, you'll need 2 teaspoons of dried apple steeped in a cup of hot water for at least 5 minutes. You can use apple blossoms to make tea and we have included a recipe specifically for peels and cores (see *page 156*).

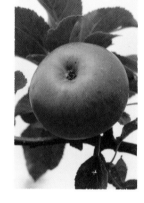

HEALTH BENEFITS

Apples have a decent number of vitamins and minerals that will ooze out into a tea. Their natural soluble fiber is also good for digestion and can even be useful for people trying to lose weight, because it makes them feel fuller than they are.

BLEND IT

Apple is excellent for adding to any fruit tea blend for some natural sweetness and fruity flavor, and it is also good with spices, such as cinnamon (see *page 122*), nutmeg, or rooty licorice brews.

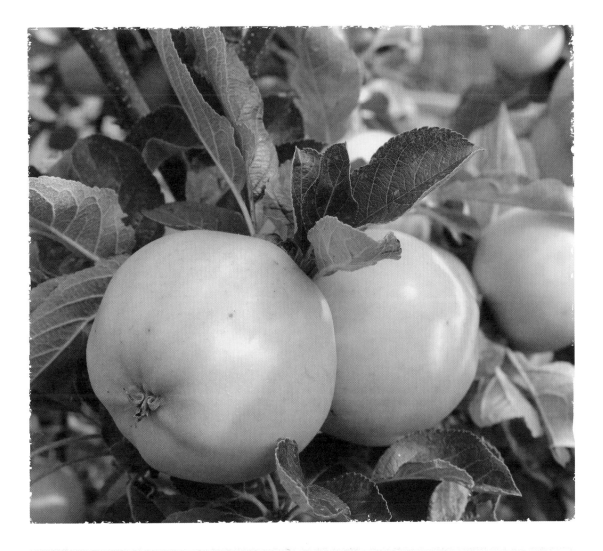

HOW TO PLANT A FRUIT TREE

1 Plant your fruit tree between November and March, when the plant is dormant.

2 Choose a sunny, preferably sheltered spot and dig a hole one-third wider than the root ball, and about 1 foot deep. Square holes are best for establishing roots—a round hole can cause the roots to spiral.

3 Hammer a support stake into the hole, making sure it sits off-center and there is room for the tree.

4 Soak the root ball thoroughly, and place in the hole. Backfill the hole and firm the soil down gently over the roots.

5 Attach a tree tie to the stake and trunk.

6 Stand back and admire your lovely tree.

7 Water the tree thoroughly and continue to water at least once a week for the first six months after planting.

Bladder Wrack

(*Fucus vesiculosus*)

Bladder wrack is a species of seaweed, easily identifiable by the small air pocket sacks positioned on its tendrils, which help it to bob up and down in the ocean. It's a common sight on rocky shorelines, where you can see it clinging to rocks like slimy Bubble Wrap. To be honest, bladder wrack tea will divide opinion. Some of you will hate it, some of you will loathe it, but bladder wrack is a seafaring superfood, packed to the gills with vitamins and minerals and is ridiculously good for you. Consider this our healthy gift to you.

FORAGE IT

If you live near the Atlantic coast, bladder wrack is best harvested from mid- to late summer when the plant is at its vitamin-packed prime. Extra caution is advised when foraging for seaweed, because there is a danger of being cut off by rising tides. Rocks festooned with seaweed can also be extremely slippery—a careless beach forager can easily be wrongfooted and end up taking an unscheduled dip in the sea, or skid over rocks and have flailing limbs rasped by a thousand knobbly barnacles. Make sure you are not harvesting your brackish bounty next to a sewage pipe.

BREW IT

Take your seaweed and wash it THOROUGHLY in fresh water. Let it dry in the sun and turn it frequently to avoid it becoming rancid. No one wants rancid seaweed tea. Grind or chop up ½–1 teaspoon dried, brittle seaweed per cup, letting it infuse in a cup of boiling water for 5 minutes.

SEAWEED FERTILIZER

Does the very thought of drinking seaweed tea disgust you? Don't worry, you can make seaweed plant fertilizer and use it to feed your plants instead. Liquid seaweed fertilizer contains many nutrients that are beneficial for plants, including nitrogen, phosphate, potassium, and magnesium, and making it is easy:

1 Wash your seaweed thoroughly to rid it of salt, sand, and seaborne debris.

2 Pile the seaweed into a bucket and top with water.

3 Place a lid on the bucket and let the seaweed steep for about a month.

4 Strain the resulting liquid into airtight containers. Just be wary of the putrid smell that will hit your nostrils when you remove the lid.

5 Add a couple of capfuls of your newly made fertilizer to a watering can and water around the bottom of your plants, being careful not to spill any on the foliage, because this may cause scorching. Store your fertilizer somewhere cool and dark, where it should keep for a month or so.

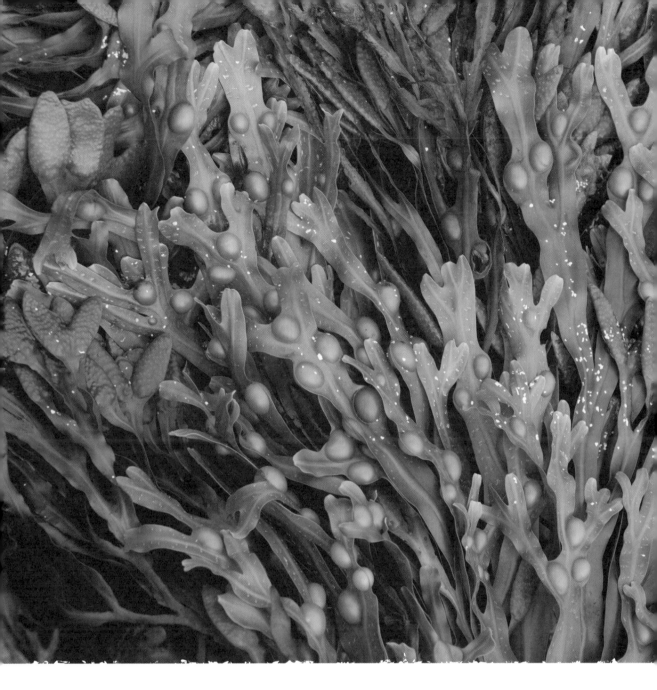

HEALTH BENEFITS

Bladder wrack is packed with healthy vitamins and minerals, including iodine, which has been extensively used to treat goiter—an unsightly swelling of the thyroid gland in the neck caused by iodine deficiency. The Romans used it to help soothe joint pains, and it's also rich in algin, which can act as a laxative.

BLEND IT

Bladder wrack tea can be difficult to stomach on its own, so add some sprigs of mint or a teaspoon of something spicy to combat its salty nature. A drop of honey or maple syrup will also help.

Bay

(Laurus nobilis)

We're real admirers of bay trees—also known as bay laurel or sweet bay*—for being one of the few exotic herbal ingredients we're able to grow with ease. Their evergreen nature also means we can rely on a year-round harvest. The leaves have a mild spiciness that is great to cook with (it's a common ingredient in garam masala) and their distinctive aroma is especially effective in hot drinks.

GROW IT

Bay is a low-maintenance plant that can be grown as a tree or a shrub, used for hedging, or constrained to a plant pot, where it's often trimmed into topiary and stuck on each side of a front door to make the house look smart. Free food pickers might also find it growing in parks and other public spaces. Be warned that there are some plants with the laurel name that are poisonous, so make sure you know what you're picking. *Laurus nobilis* is the most familiar of the culinary bay laurels to look for.

BREW IT

You can brew a simple bay leaf tea with 3–4 fresh or dried leaves. Put them in a saucepan with enough water for your chosen mug, bring to a boil, and simmer for 5 minutes. Let cool before straining, and drink on its own, with a slice of lemon, or a splash of milk. You can also crumble dried leaves into blends—this works particularly well in chai teas.

HEALTH BENEFITS

Bay leaves have a long list of vitamins and reported health benefits that range from anti-inflammatory properties to curing dandruff. The comforting spicy aromas of bay leaf oil are also popular with aromatherapists,** and bay is commonly used for arthritic aches and pains.

BLEND IT

Its subtly spicy aromas and flavors lend themselves well to spiced teas and chais (see *page 130*).

---

* *Not to be confused with sweet bay that is a type of magnolia.*

** *Those spicy aromas are less popular with bugs; bay leaf oil is often a feature of insect repellents.*

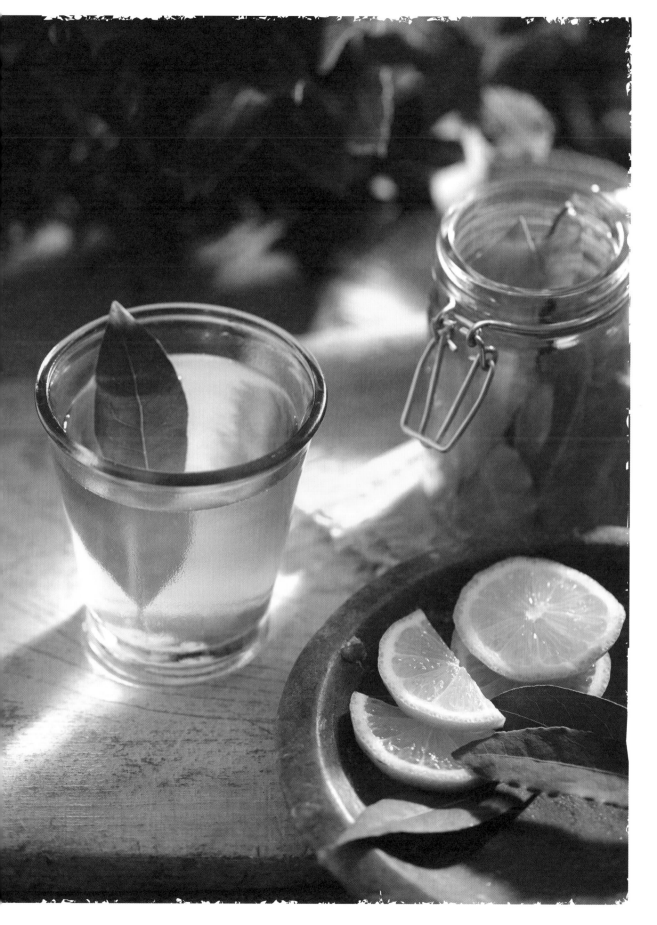

Sage

(Salvia officinalis)

We had our doubts about sage as a tea ingredient, because its strong savory flavor has such an association with stuffing we couldn't imagine drinking it. However, it turns out that sage tea tastes great, giving us another reason to regularly pick leaves and peg back the rampaging plants in our garden patches.

GROW IT

We've always found sage a hit-and-miss plant. Sometimes it struggles to muster the strength to get established, but try it in a different location and it thrives, rambling over a vast area and smothering anything in its path. Sage is a member of the mint family and there are hundreds of cultivars and wild varieties: some annual, some perennial, some flowering and with leaves in every shade of green you can imagine (and purple or gold). Unfortunately, not all of these are edible, so choose the common sage, *Salvia officinalis*.

BREW IT

Try infusing 6–8 fresh leaves, or 2 teaspoons of dried leaves per cup of hot water. Besides its savory herb flavors, it also has some bitterness that we think makes it extra tea-worthy.

HEALTH BENEFITS

Ancient Egyptians used sage to aid fertility, but these days it's most commonly known as a potential antioxidant. Some people also believe it can help to reduce anxiety and lower cholesterol. It's a common ingredient in supplements designed to support women going through menopause.

BLEND IT

Our sage advice is to drink it on its own, but you could try adding lemon or a few warming spices, such as cinnamon, bay, or cloves.

DID YOU KNOW?

For a spectacular member of the *Salvia* family, take a look at the bright red flowers of the pineapple sage (or scarlet pineapple), a Mexican native that does indeed smell of pineapple.

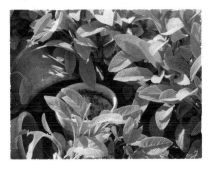

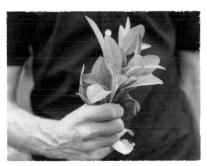

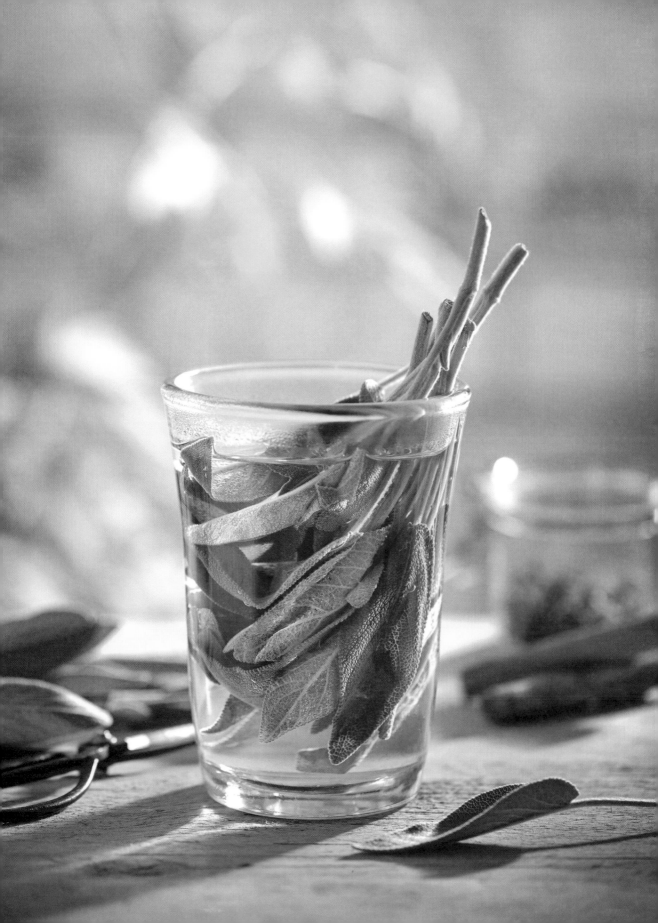

Borage
(Borago officinalis)

This hairy, hardy annual hails from the Mediterranean, but it has managed to find a foothold and flourish in parts of North America, thanks to its tolerance of a variety of soil conditions and climates. If you have the space, borage is a handy herb to have growing in your garden borders. Use it as a companion plant, because it will attract a wide variety of pollinating insects, which find the striking blue flower heads irresistible. Its leaves also happen to make a tasty, healthy tea. Just be warned—bees love borage so much you may well have to fight them for it.

FORAGE IT
Look for borage in pastures and in deciduous woodland. Its large leaves are similar to other, more unpalatable species, but its star-shape flowers, which hang in downward-facing clusters, are distinctive and start to appear from early summer.

GROW IT
Borage is easy to grow from seed and prefers a site in the sun in poor, sandy soil. Make sure you sow it in its final position—it has a long tap root and doesn't respond well to being dug up and moved. Deadheading the flowers will help promote new buds throughout the summer. Borage also grows well in plant pots, but make sure you stake the plants, because they have a tendency to flop when unsupported.

BREW IT
Coarsely chop a small handful of fresh leaves, put them into a cup, and cover

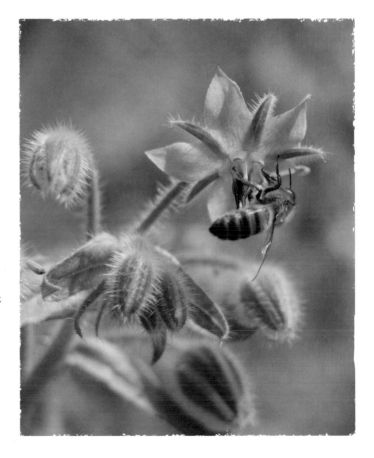

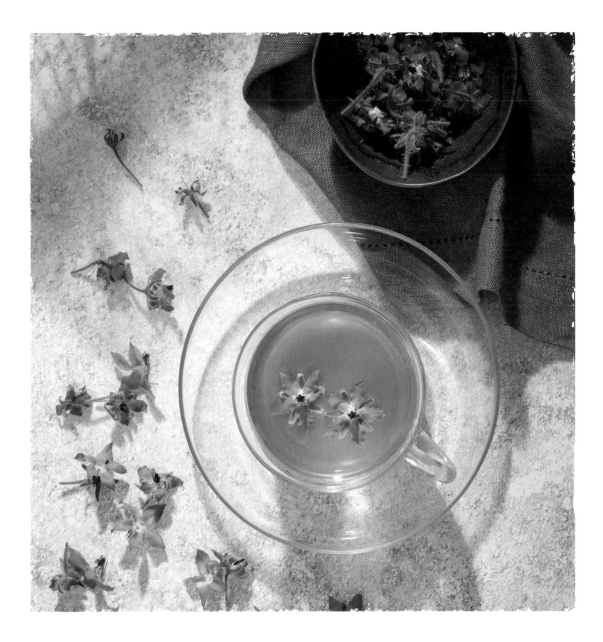

with boiling water. Let infuse for 5–10 minutes, then strain, serve, and sip your subtly tannic tea.

HEALTH BENEFITS

Both the flowers and leaves of borage, as well as the oil from its seeds, are used extensively in herbal medicine to treat gastrointestinal disorders. Borage is also used as a treatment for colds and lung infections. In Arabic, borage is called "the father of sweat," which alludes to the plant's diaphoretic properties.

BLEND IT

Try blending a few leaves with other herb-flavor brews and use the blue flowers as a garnish for making fancy-looking iced teas.

Cherry

(Prunus)

In his collection of acclaimed pastoral poems, A. E. Housman described the cherry as the "loveliest of trees." King Henry VIII of England thought so too—on a trip to Flanders he was so captivated by its handsome visage and tasty fruit that he ordered the planting of England's first cherry orchard in Kent. We are also big fans, because the cherry happens to be a versatile caddy ally. You can make a tea from the bark, stems, and blossoms, and the fruit can be squeezed into splendid syrups for the loveliest of teas.

FORAGE IT

Search and locate cherry trees in springtime by looking for the emerging clusters of white or pink cup-shape flowers in woodland and pasture. Make a note of the location, so you can get in quick when the fruit matures and before birds raid your intended stash. There are a few different species you may stumble across when out foraging: cherry plum (*Prunus cerasifera*), bird cherry (*Prunus padus*), sour cherry (*Prunus cerasus*), and sweet cherry (*Prunus avium*). You may also see ornamental cherry trees growing in parks, but remember that foraging in local parks isn't strictly foraging—it's kind of stealing—so always seek permission first before you start shaking the branches for your tea-making experiments.

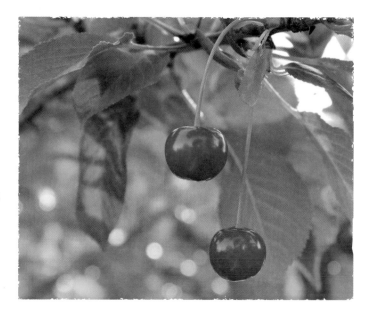

cherries require pollination partners in order to produce fruit, so you may need to plant a pollinating pal.

GROW IT

Planting a cherry is easy, just follow the tried-and-tested fruit tree method (see *page 93*). Cherry trees come in sweet and sour species. The sweet

BREW THE STEMS

To make cherry stem tea, take a handful of cherries, remove the fruit, then dry out the stems, either on a warm windowsill or in a dehydrator.

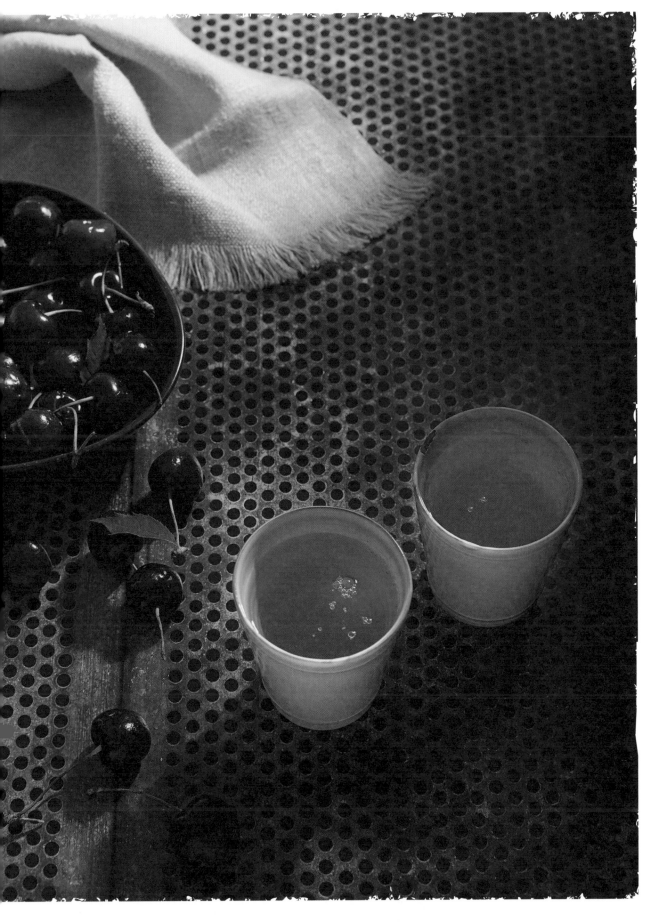

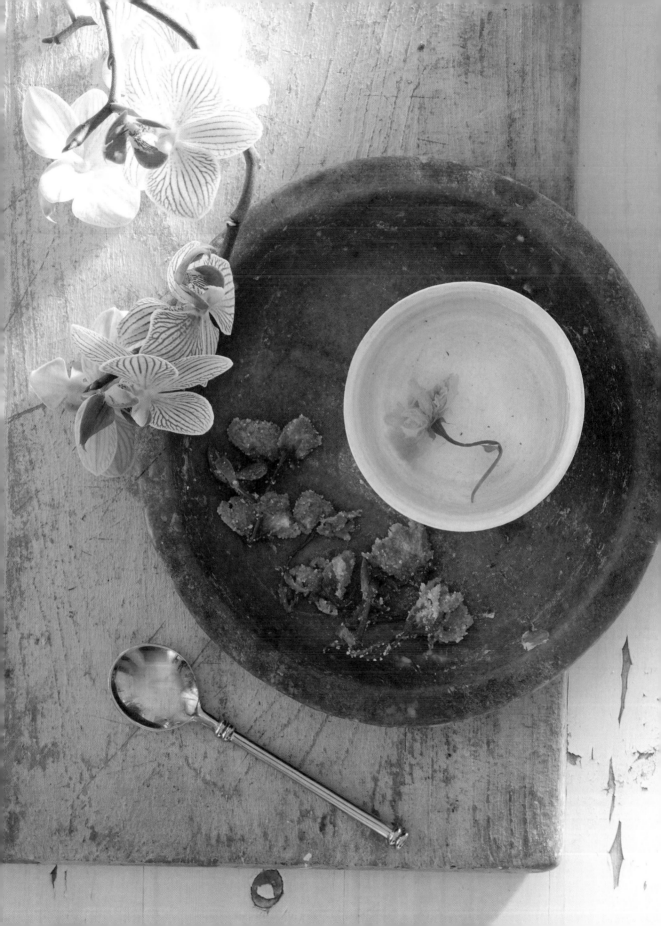

HOW TO PICKLE CHERRY BLOSSOMS TO MAKE SAKURA TEA

1 Gather 2 cups of pink blossoms in springtime, just as they are emerging.

2 Combine with 2 teaspoons of salt and refrigerate for 2–3 days.

3 Press the blossoms with a paper towel to remove excess moisture, then cover with ¼ cup plum vinegar and let marinate for an additional 3 days.

4 Drain off the vinegar and allow the blossoms to dry before storing in a jam jar packed with salt.

5 To make Sakura Tea, put 3–4 of the salted, pickled blossoms into a cup and pour over boiling water.

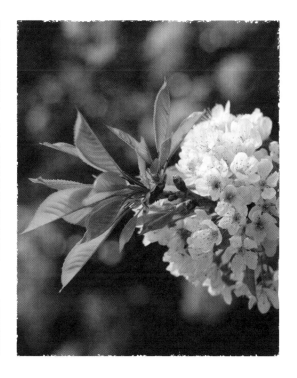

Take a healthy pinch of dried stems, drop them in a cup, add boiling water, and let steep for 10 minutes. Strain, then serve for a delicate, lightly tannic brew.

BREW THE FRUIT

Turn the stemless cherries into syrups for making fruity brews, such as our Blackberry Frappé (see *page 172*).

BREW THE BARK

Wild cherry bark tea is supposedly good for soothing coughs. A slither of bark should be chopped and dried before adding a couple of teaspoons to a mug of boiling water. It makes for a pretty astringent woody-tasting brew (unsurprisingly), so it needs to be blended with other more palatable cup buddies. Try smoothing those rough edges with a healthy dose of mint.

BREW THE BLOSSOM

The fruit of ornamental species, such as the Japanese cherry (*Prunus serrulata*) tend to be too sharp to be used in syrups without adding industrial levels of sugar to balance out the acidity. Instead, gather their blossoms in springtime and attempt to make a salty, umami Sakura Tea (see above).

HEALTH BENEFITS

Cherry stem tea has been used in the treatment of inflammation of the bladder. It's also deemed to be a pretty effective laxative. Go careful now.

BLEND IT

Anyone with a penchant for fruity pies knows that cherry goes well with cinnamon, so add 1 or 2 pinches to your syrup or cherry stem tea. Loose leaf black tea also tastes great with the addition of a few drops of cherry syrup.

WARNING!

Some parts of cherries, in particular, the pits (like those of apricots, almonds, peaches, and plums), contain small amounts of cyanide. Although you would have to ingest a lot for it to have an effect, drink all cherry-base teas in moderation.

Licorice

(Glycyrrhiza glabra)

The licorice plant possesses one of the tastiest roots around with a depth of flavor few other ingredients can match. Besides its obvious similarity to anise, it has an addictive earthy quality and so much sweetness it actually tastes juicy. And there's even more good news for wild tea brewers—it's a healthy tonic, too.

GROW IT

Licorice's dream environment is a warm spot on the bank of a river or stream. To try growing your own, if you live in a warm region, give it your sunniest spot in well-draining, ideally sandy soil. Seeds are difficult to germinate, and young plants are vulnerable to cold, so protect them from frost for a few years before planting outside.

Once established, and given the right conditions, the plant will develop a long tap root and rhizomes that can spread to cover a large area. To harvest, dig up the plant in late fall and cut away the roots, leaving the crown intact. You'll then need to nurture the crown through winter by storing it in compost somewhere cool and dark before planting outside again in spring. If this sounds like too much work, then dried roots are readily available for culinary purposes.

BREW IT

To get the full flavors of licorice in a tea, you're better off decocting the root. Cut off a piece about 2 inches long, split it lengthwise, and mash it gently with a mortar and pestle, then simmer for a minimum of 10 minutes in enough boiling water for your mug plus an extra third for evaporation. Chopping and grinding makes it suitable for steeping, with a pinch or two of the resulting powder adding its rich, flavorsome notes to tea blends.

HEALTH BENEFITS

Licorice roots contain hundreds of different chemical compounds, and the list of potential health benefits from these is vast. Scientists have been busily studying the root to ascertain its healing capabilities in many areas, including skin conditions, stomach pains, cough treatments, hepatitis C, and tooth decay.* Despite all this potential goodness, licorice also contains toxins that can cause health problems if taken in excess.

BLEND IT

You'll find licorice sneaking into a lot of caffeine-free, commercially available teas, where it adds complexity to many flavor combinations. Try it with leafy brews to give them some depth of flavor and a natural sweetness.

DID YOU KNOW?

The Dutch and Norwegians love licorice-flavored candies, some of which are mixed with salty-tasting ammonium chloride and are known as *salmiak*. It is an acquired taste, but one that is worth persevering with.

* *However, regularly eating licorice candies will almost certainly encourage tooth decay.*

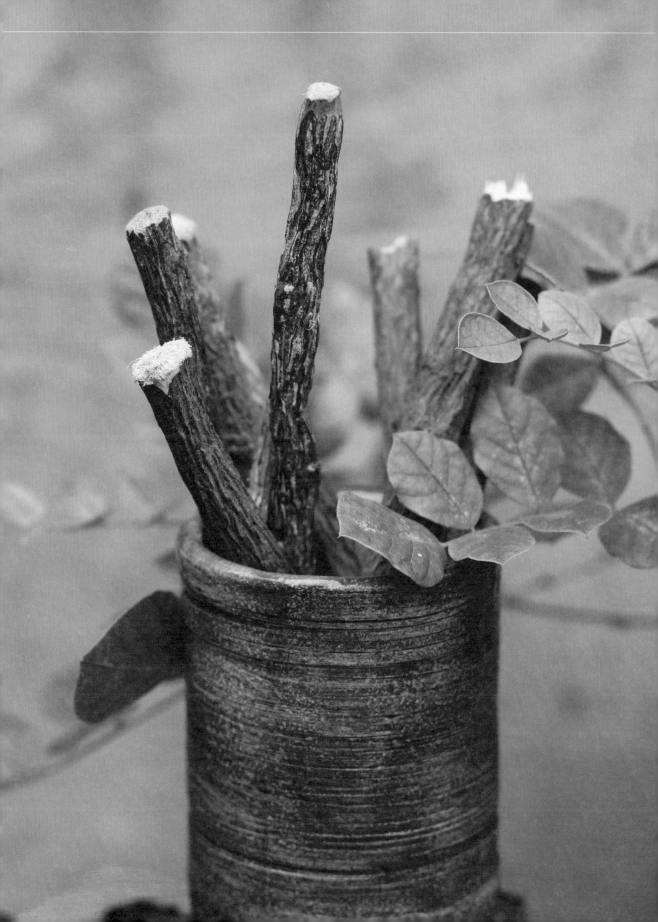

Lemongrass

(Cymbopogon citratus)

A hero of Thai cooking, lemongrass has sweet, aromatic lemon flavors that add a freshness to food and drinks without the acidic tang of its citrusy namesake. You can use both leaves and stalks to make tea, with the latter doubling up as a handy stirring implement.

GROW IT

Lemongrass can be a little difficult to grow away from the tropical parts of the world it favors. Nick once kept a plant alive for two years before it perished, either through lack of heat, humidity, or incorrect watering. Healthy, longer-living lemongrass plants can grow into huge, grassy clumps. Only a few of the fifty-plus lemongrass cultivars are used for cooking, so if you try to grow your own, be certain it's edible.

BREW IT

You can use the stalks (2 stalks per cup, outer layer removed and mashed to release their flavor), but you'll get much more from steeping the leaves (1 teaspoon per cup) in a cup of boiling water for 5 minutes. Both parts can also be dried. Try lemongrass on its own or with black tea, serve hot or cold, and give it some extra zest with a lime garnish.

HEALTH BENEFITS

There are countless health claims surrounding lemongrass, from the

TURN STALKS INTO PLANTS

You can grow your own lemongrass plants from store-bought stalks, if they have some of the bottom end still intact. Simply remove any loose or dry outer layers, put them into a jar of water, and fill to cover the lower third of the stalks. Refresh the water every few days and eventually roots will appear. When you have a healthy nest of small roots, put the stalks into a plant pot filled with potting mix (you can stick several stalks in one pot and grow as a clump) and keep indoors until established.

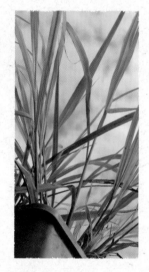

relief of anxiety to the prevention of infections, but we can't find much in the way of proven benefits. It features regularly in Ayurvedic health brews and is popular for medicinal teas in Brazil, where it's often paired with pineapple.

BLEND IT

Lemongrass blends well with other fruity and spicy flavors, such as apple, ginger, and cinnamon.

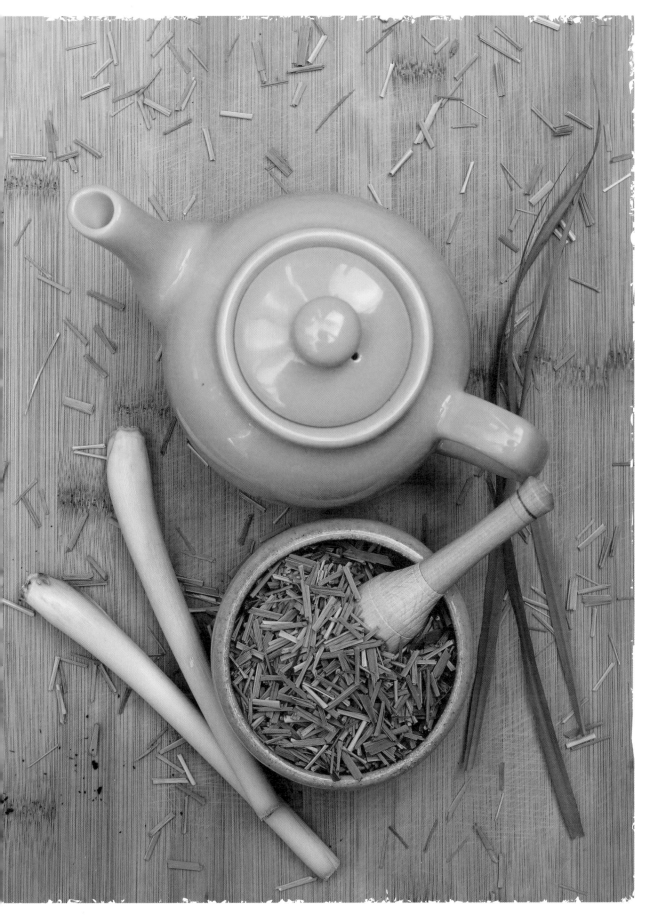

Beet

(Beta vulgaris)

The beet has enjoyed a long history of culinary and medicinal use. Evidence of beet cultivation can be traced back to Neolithic times, and the ancient Greeks were avid growers (but they ate the leaves, not the roots). The Romans were especially fond of beet, and the plant features heavily in the Apicius manuscript. After a hard day marching around in uncomfortable sandals, they would often cheer themselves with a carafe or two of wine and a nice beet salad. The Romans never really took to drinking tea, but we think they've missed out—when it comes to making tasty, vegetable-base beverages, this bulbous, ruddy root is hard to beet.

GROW IT

Beets are one of the easiest vegetables to grow, making them a favorite in our garden. They prefer to grow in well-drained soil and will thrive in fertile conditions, so if you can, dig in some well-rotted manure prior to planting. Harvest beets when the roots are the size of golf balls, because that's when they are at their most flavorsome.

BREW IT

Beets make a fine brew, hot or iced. It's a good idea to wear gloves during preparation, because this ruddy-hued root will stain your hands crimson, making it look like you've been party to some kind of gruesome crime.*

For a hot, tasty chai, grate ½ beet into a cup, then add a couple of pinches of grated ginger. Top the cup with boiling water, cover it with a saucer, and let steep for 10–15 minutes. To serve, add a squeeze of lemon juice and 1 teaspoon of honey.

For an iced beet tea, follow the directions above, but let it cool completely before straining and pouring over ice. Add a couple of sprigs of mint for a fresh summer flourish.

HEALTH BENEFITS

Studies have shown that eating beets can significantly lower blood pressure and fight heart disease. It is also believed to increase libido, working in a similar way to Viagra by increasing nitric oxide levels in the body and increasing blood flow to your nether regions.

BLEND IT

Besides making a crimson-color chai (see above), you can use dried beet in healthy tonics, and it pairs well with sweet apple (see Harvest Brew *page 128*).

DID YOU KNOW?

Garlic breath can be nullified by a glass of beet juice. We've yet to come across a vegetable that nullifies beet breath.

* *If you were unimpressed by the results of our lemon tea recipes on page 88, you could always use them as a handwash; lemon juice can help remove beet stains from hands.*

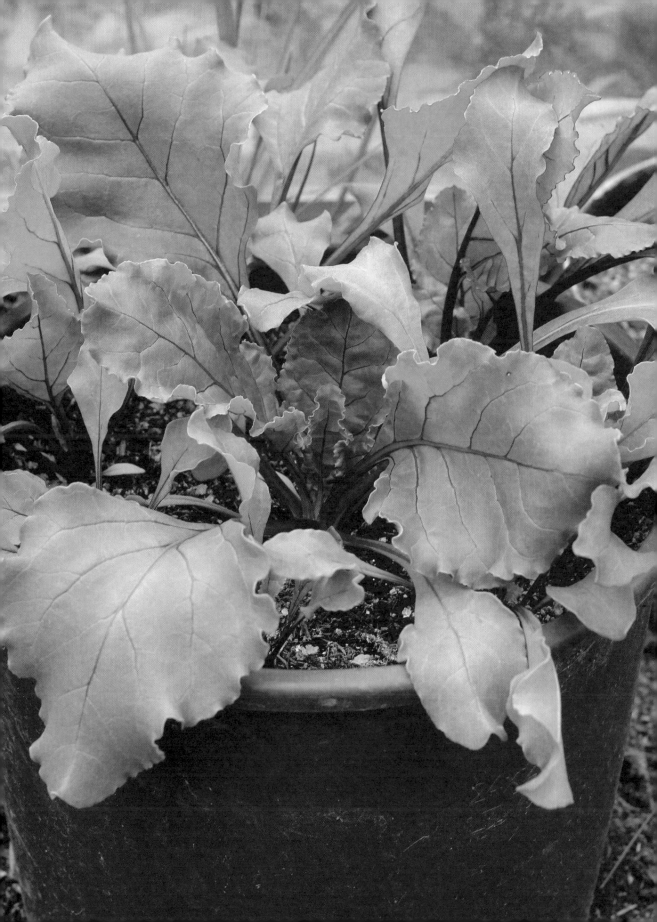

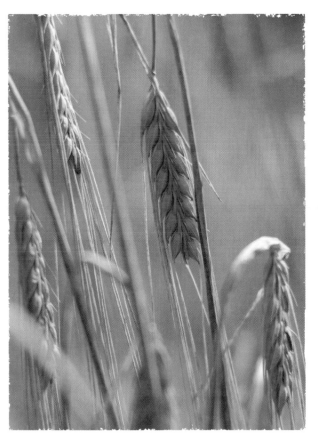
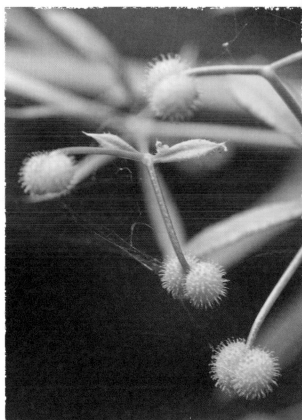
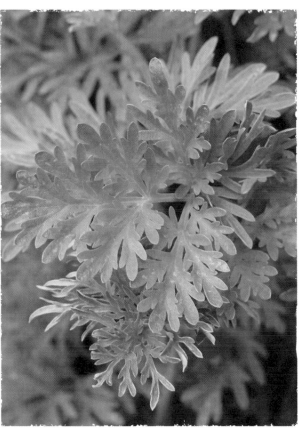
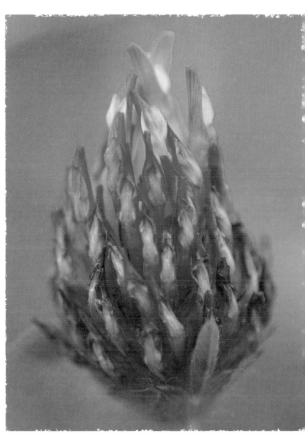

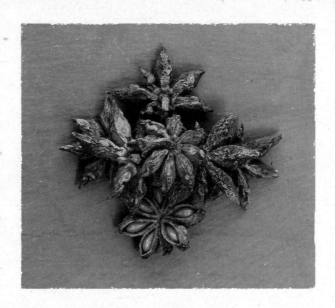

Best of the Rest

In this section, we feature even more of our favorite ingredients, chosen for their brewing greatness or because of the teatime tales they can tell.

ACORNS

The small nuts from the mighty oak can be roasted to make coffee (see *page 169*).

ANISE

The seeds of this Mediterranean plant are used in many candies and boozes, including ouzo, absinthe, arak, sambuca, and pastis. They also impart a sweet licorice-like flavor to tea blends. Lightly crush a teaspoonful before adding to hot water. In Holland, an anise-flavored, milky brew called *anijsmelk* is popular. Simply add 1 teaspoon of anise to a mug of milk and heat in a saucepan. When it reaches boiling point, turn down the heat and simmer for 5 minutes. Strain into a mug and stir in 2 teaspoons of honey for sweetness.

ANISE HYSSOP

This perennial herb is neither anise nor hyssop. However, it does have a minty taste similar to hyssop with a sprinkling of anise flavor and therefore is great to grow for teas.

BANANA

There has been a recent trend for boiling banana peel to make a pre-bed tea that can supposedly help you sleep. It's not for us and, because bananas receive a lot of chemical spraying, anyone eager to try it should make sure their fruit is organic. Dried bananas yield little flavor when infused, yet 3–4 crushed slices in a cup make a surprisingly enjoyable drink, with just a whisper of banana sweetness emerging.

BARLEY

This cereal crop is grown for beer, whiskey, and Roasted Barley Tea (see *page 144*).

BASIL

About 5 medium fresh sweet basil leaves (*Ocimum basilicum*) make a tea with a tasty tingle; the herb also complements some fruity brews. Even better is lemon basil (*Ocimum basilicum* var. *citriodorum*), which has the added benefit of punchy lemony notes.

BERGAMOT

A citrus fruit that's a little like a sour orange and is used to flavor Earl Grey tea.

BLACK PEPPER

A pinch of pepper does wonders for warming up a cup of tea and is useful in spiced beverages.

BURDOCK

In the UK, we're familiar with the use of burdock as a double act with dandelion in a soft drink, and the two also used to team up in ancient meads and beers. Burdock's seeds have hooks, which easily attach to clothes and have been claimed to be the inspiration for the invention of Velcro, but it's the unusual mild, earthy flavor of the roots that are responsible for the plant's use in cooking and tea making.

BAMBOO

While the shoots of bamboo are commonly used in Chinese cooking, it's the young leaves of some cultivars that are used for tea. Apparently, they're rich in silica, which is claimed to promote hair growth and, because we've never seen a bald panda, who are we to disagree?

BLUEBERRY / BILBERRY

Both leaves and berries are suitable for tea making, with the latter making a colorful addition to fruity blends. If you can't find them in the wild, grow them at home in acidic soil—ours are confined to plant pots and in fall we race the birds to pick them. Their smooth skins are good at holding in the juice, so cut them in half for speedier drying. Confusingly, "blueberry tea" is also the name of a cocktail that doesn't contain blueberries.

CARAWAY

Also known as Persian cumin and meridian fennel, these seeds are a common flavoring in rye bread. They have a milder anise flavor than fennel and are earthier, with a slight peppery warmth.

CARROT

Russians like a wild tea—they have been known to blend carrot greens with black tea and sometimes used dried carrots as a tea substitute during World War II.

CARDAMOM

The seed pods from two types of cardamom are used as a spice: green cardamom, which comes from the Indian plant species *Elettaria cardomomum*, and the

Himalyan black cardamom, which comes from *Amomum subulatum*. The green pods are commonly used in teas and are an essential ingredient of traditional masala chais (see *page 130*).

CASSAVA

A rooty crop from which tapioca is extracted (see Bubble Tea on *page 162*).

CATNIP

This member of the mint family makes a decent, minty-tasting tea with a slight hint of citrus. Use 1–2 teaspoons of dried flowers per cup. Cat-owning home-based workers should avoid perching a glass of catnip tea beside their laptop for obvious reasons.

CHICORY

The roasted roots make a good coffee substitute (see *page 169*).

CHILI PEPPER

Choose a cultivar that's easy to grow in your garden or on a windowsill, and use it fresh or dried to add a kick to hot drinks, such as chai (see *page 130*).

CINNAMON

The inner bark of the cinnamon tree plays a supporting role in several of our teas, delivering a warming, feel-good presence to every nostril its aroma meets. It is the essence of the festive season and can work its magic on just about any tea around. We prefer to use sticks instead of ground powder, which can be dropped into decoctions whole or crumbled into

blends. For a solo cinnamon tea, try simmering 1 stick in a mug's worth of water for 5 minutes.

CLEAVERS

The small round seeds that have a habit of sticking to your clothes can be roasted for an excellent alternative to coffee (see *page 169*).

CLOVES

These spicy little sticks are actually dried flower buds from the Indonesian clove tree. They're used in sweet and savory dishes and are often in demand at Christmas, when they're added to all kinds of mulled beverages, including winter-warming teas.

COCONUT

Coconut flavoring often appears in commercial teas, chocolates, coffee blends, and syrups, but we use it most as a milk substitute.

COMMON MALLOW

We sowed and nurtured some common mallow plants (*Mallow sylvestris*), because their leaves and flowers were reputed to make a decent, healthy tea. The results were revolting, so we won't bother again.

CORNFLOWER

Cornflower's bright blue petals are often added to tea blends, notably Earl Grey, mainly to liven their appearance with a touch of color.

CRANBERRY

These tart little berries work as well in teas as they do in festive

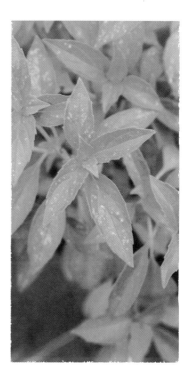

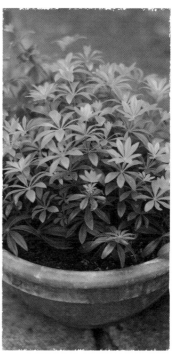

Above from top: lemon basil, sweet woodruff.

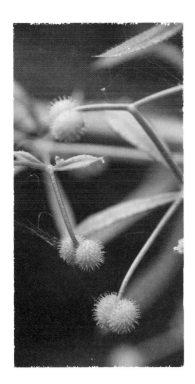

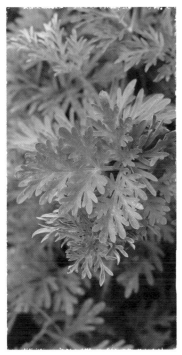

sauces. They are best in blends that feature sweeter fruits, with orange providing a common partner. Like blueberries, they're a plant that requires acidic soil—home-growers can also benefit from picking leaves for tea making.

CUCUMBER

A member of the Cucurbitaceae family, which also includes melons, squashes, and pumpkins, the cucumber is loved for its cooling character, making it popular for iced teas (see *page 158*).

EPAZOTE

This native of Central America and Mexico is a member of the goosefoot family and is so revered for its tea that it's also known as Jesuit's tea and Mexican tea. It also goes by the name stink weed and has the translated name skunk sweat. because it emits an aroma like a filthy truck leaking fuel. We read that it tastes better than it smells, but it doesn't. We grow a plant in a container, because one of the chemicals responsible for the stench (ascaridole) can also inhibit the growth of nearby plants. It has been used to kill parasites in humans and pets, and Mexicans reckon it can help reduce bloating and any resulting flatulence, so often serve it with beans—but go easy, because it's toxic and could induce vomiting or far worse.

FEVERFEW

Drinking feverfew tea was once believed to give the drinker fewer fevers, but now its most common use is in preventing migraines. It's a member of the daisy family and has strong-scented leaves not dissimilar in flavor to sage. Steep 3 leaves (fresh or dried) in a cup full of hot water for 2–3 minutes for a delicately soothing brew.

GRASS CLIPPINGS

Nope.

GROUND IVY

Low-lying *Glechoma hederacea* is a member of the mint family and can be found at the edges of fields and ditches or creeping into the corners of unweeded yards. It has dainty blue flowers and its green leaves can become tinged with purple, depending on the nutritional content of the soil it roots in. Use 6–8 fresh leaves picked in spring (or 1 teaspoon of dried leaves) for a tea that has a sagelike herbiness with a minty tingle and peppery bitterness. These flavors make it a useful hop substitute for beer, hence its alternative name—alehoof. It's not to everyone's taste, but we like it and think it works well in mint and anise blends.

HIMALAYAN BALSAM

In order to help eradicate this invasive riverbank menace, we'd love to be able to say that Himalayan balsam makes a lovely brew. We can't. The best we can suggest is that you can freeze its (admittedly handsome) flowers into ice cubes and then float them in a nice iced tea (see *pages 154 and 158*).

JASMINE

The blossoms of the common jasmine (*Jasminum officinale*), or the national flower of the Philippines (*Jasminum sambac*), are blended with other teas, most commonly green, to produce the popular aromatic jasmine tea. The tea is often sold as "pearls"—rolled up green tea leaves that have been infused with jasmine's fragrance.

LIME

Lime's main function in Western drinks is as a garnishing alternative to lemon. We think it deserves more attention than that and happily use it in cold teas for some sour fruitiness (see Tropical Hibiscus Sun Tea, *page 149*).

In Arabian countries, it takes even more of the limelight (pun intended) and a popular tea is made from the dried fruits (commonly called *limu Omani*, because the drying method originated in Oman). You'll need 1 lime per cup (add another half for a large mug) broken into chunks and simmered in a cup's worth of water for 5 minutes before serving and sweetening to taste.

MARSHMALLOW

The roots from this wild perennial were the original flavoring ingredient for the candy favored by amateur campfire chefs. They also crop up in tea blends that promote relaxation and calmness.

MUGWORT

This wild cousin to wormwood can be used as an alternative to its more bitter relative.

OLIVE LEAF

Dried olive leaves make a tea that is rich in vitamins and antioxidants. It can take a while for the flavors to completely seep out, so steep for as long as you can. You'll be rewarded with a silky, mellow brew that has a unique flavor verging on fishiness, but try not to let that put you off, because it's better than it sounds.

ORANGE

This much enjoyed citrus fruit can be useful to add some sweet juicy flavors to blends and is a winning choice for chocolaty drinks (see *page 128*).

PUZZLEWEED

Alas, there is no such plant as the puzzleweed. It is here simply to make sure that everyone reading this is paying attention.

RED CLOVER

Red clover can be found dotted around fields in early summer, nodding its fluffy pink heads among the swathes of green grass. These flowers make a pleasant cup of tea and you only need 4–5 fresh heads per mug. The tea is delicate and, therefore, hard to describe—we're going with a faintly sweet melonish aroma and a dry, haylike flavor. And if you're hoping you'll be sipping on a pink or red brew, then you're out of luck—the hot water will make it turn a vivid lime green.

RHUBARB

This vegetable thinks it's a fruit. It combines excellently with ginger (see *page 167* for more).

ROOIBOS

Rooibos (or red bush) is a rugged, broom-like plant that grows in the Cederberg region of South Africa. Its needle-shape leaves are oxidized and made into a caffeine-free tea that has a sweet, nutty taste. When asking for it in smart tea establishments, you should pronounce it "roy-boss" to demonstrate your exemplary tea knowledge, thanks to reading this book.

SCENTED GERANIUMS

Confusingly, scented geraniums of the *Pelargonium* genus are not the same as geraniums, which is the name of another plant group and not something you want to use in your beverages. To mark their difference, they're known as scented geraniums on account of their strong aromas.

To be sure you're dealing with something both edible and tasty, choose a scented geranium, such as the daintily pink-flowered cultivar "Attar of Roses," which has a heady rosy fragrance that is much admired by perfumers and dessert makers.

The best way to get these flavors into a tea, coffee, cake, or pastry is by making a scented sugar from scented geranium leaves. Finely chop 3 leaves, mix them into ½ cup of sugar, and seal in a jar for 24 hours before opening.

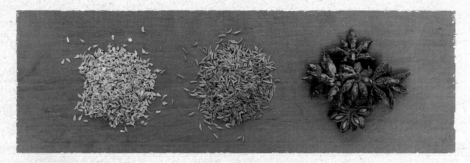

Left: anise, caraway, star anise.

Opposite, clockwise from top-left: ground ivy, cornflower, epazote, feverfew, scented geranium.

STAR ANISE

A popular Chinese spice that tastes like its namesake, anise, and looks like a star. See *page 151* for its star brewing qualities.

STEVIA

This sweet-leaved Brazilian native is seen as a miracle sugar replacement by some and a mysterious evil by others—it has even been banned in some countries. We've made several unsuccessful attempts to grow it from seed (germination is tricky), so bought an established plant instead. The leaves should be picked before flowering and, although we've heard that some plants fail to deliver sweetness, ours has it in great abundance.

SWEET WOODRUFF

Also known as *Waldmeister* and wild baby's breath, this ground-hugging herb can be seen growing in yards and in dappled woodland shade. Dry out the leaves and steep them in hot water for a floral brew that smells like freshly mown hay—the longer you steep, the more fragrant your tea will be. Flick over to *page 166* for our woodruff syrup recipe.

THYME

This herb is disappointing in the tea-making department, with an oily flavor that doesn't suit hot drinks. However, it is worth growing for soups and stews, and so you can make "tea-thyme" jokes (not that we'd stoop so low).

TULSI

Looks a little like basil, tastes a little like basil, makes a tea a little like basil, and is also called holy basil. But it's a different plant to the more well-known culinary basil. We've found it a little less reliable to grow than sweet basil but, if you want to add some color to your greenhouse, it's worth trying a purple-leaved cultivar.

TURMERIC

Turmeric root is a common favorite of Asian dishes and has recently been transformed into a star beverage ingredient, lending its glorious golden hue to whatever dish it's added to. The turmeric plant is a relative of ginger and prefers to grow in the hot and wet parts of India and Asia. Simmer 1–2 teaspoons in water to make a tea or turn to *page 142* for our version of the popular turmeric latte.

VALERIAN

The roots of common valerian (*Valeriana officinalis*, not to be confused with other plants with the valerian moniker) have long been used as a tea for insomniacs, and it cuddles up with other sleepy ingredients in Sue's Hop to Bed brew (see *page 126*). In medieval times, the plants were tucked into Swedish grooms' wedding clothes to see off jealous elves.

WORMWOOD

This attractive, silvery-green-leaf perennial is a good looker in flower-borders and is sometimes known as absinthium, green ginger, madder wort, or bitter hellion. The leaves of the species *Artemisia absinthium* have a powerfully bitter flavor and are used in absinthe, vermouth, and herbal liqueurs. Thujone is present in the leaves and is said to be one of the chemicals responsible for absinthe's notoriety as a mind-bending booze. Wormwood is also used as a medicinal tea, most commonly to treat intestinal problems, and is mixed with green tea in Morocco as an alternative to mint.

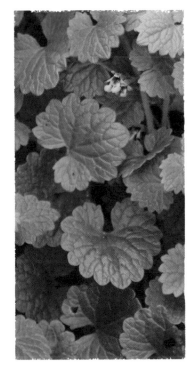
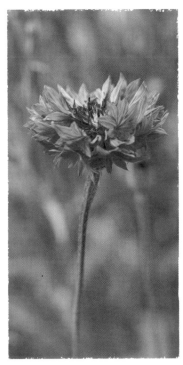
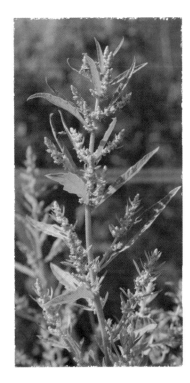
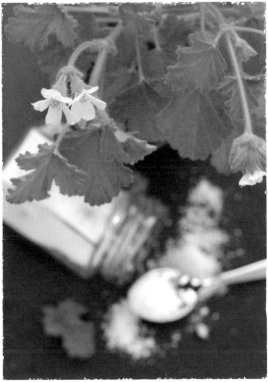
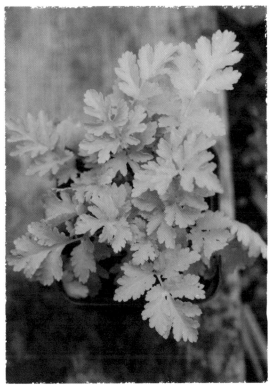

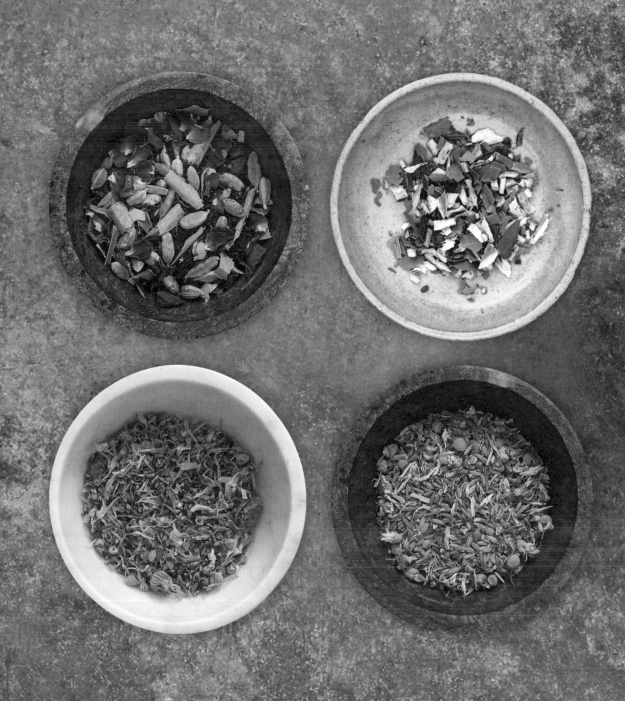

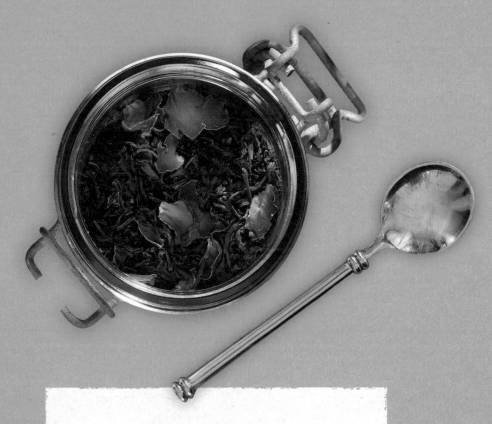

Blends

To be a true wild tea master, you've got to
blend. Mixing together different dried tea
ingredients lets you create a whole range
of flavor combinations that you can store
and dip into for an instant brew whenever
the mood strikes.

PERFECT PARTNERS

To set you on the path to blending brilliance, here are some of our favorite double acts. Try playing around with the proportions of each ingredient to get a feeling for how the flavors work in combination with each other and, if you're feeling in an experimental mood, introduce a third flavor to build a more uniquely complex blend.

MINT AND LEMON

You can pair mint or lemon with just about any other ingredient in this book and strike a winning combination, so it's no surprise that they relish each other's company. We like our mint with a hint of lemon and, for all the more complicated blends and recipes in this book, it's a tea that is hard to beat.

Serve: 2 teaspoons per cup
3 parts dried mint leaves
1 part dried lemon peel

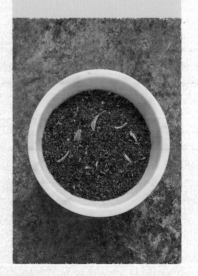

RHUBARB AND GINGER

Rhubarb is one of many foods that claims to be ginger's best friend. There's something about ginger's zingy warmth that makes the tart pink stalks from our unruly garden-dwelling rhubarb seem faintly exotic. Before drying rhubarb, slice it into pencil-thick strips, and it will soon shrivel into string, making it easy to break into your tea blend. Garnish with an orange wheel to bring out the vegetable's fruitier side.

Serve: 1 teaspoon per cup
1 part dried ginger
1 part dried rhubarb
1 orange wheel, to garnish (optional)

APPLE AND CINNAMON

Baked apples are always improved by a pinch of cinnamon, and you can re-create that comforting autumnal combination in tea form.

Serve: 2 teaspoons per cup
3 parts dried apple
2 parts cinnamon stick

Crumble a cinnamon stick with small chunks of dried apple and infuse for a good 10 minutes (or simmer in a saucepan if you don't mind the extra cleaning up). Apple is naturally sweet, but if you crave more sweetness, add some brown sugar.

A NOTE ON QUANTITIES

The quantities in this section are based on the volume of dried ingredients when crumbled, chopped, or ground. We've measured them as proportional "parts" so you can decide on your own quantities. For example, if you're making an initial small experimental batch, then make each "part" a teaspoon; for larger batches, each part can be measured out in a larger volume. For each of these blends, infuse in hot water for 5 minutes unless otherwise stated.

THREE OF A KIND

When coming up with combinations of three or more ingredients, it can help to narrow down the choice by thinking of things that naturally go together. This could be anything from ingredients that have a similar flavor, to plants that share the same season, or even those that grow together. Here we've taken inspiration from our own garden, a trip to the coast and the tea-friendly flavors of lemon...

WILD GARDEN TEA

Being lazy gardeners, we'll use any excuse to avoid the hard labor of weeding, so we're grateful that some of the plants that have bullied their way into our yards make excellent teas. This blend is a combination of three favorite wild plants that others consider weeds—so dodge the digging, hang up your hoes, and get to work on this wholesome brew instead.

Serve: 2 teaspoons per cup
5 parts dried dandelion flowers
3 parts dried nettle leaves
3 parts dried yarrow leaves

THREE WAYS WITH LEMON

Have you noticed how smart modern chefs like to show off their range of culinary skills by serving up the same ingredient in three different ways? This is our liquid antidote to such nonsense—a tea made with three ingredients that all taste of lemon. To compliment the zesty lemon of the actual fruit, we've introduced the sweet flavors of lemon verbena and the calming herbal notes of lemon balm. Three lemons, one great tea.

Serve: 1 teaspoon per cup
2 parts dried lemon verbena leaves
1 part dried lemon balm leaves
1 part dried lemon peel

COASTAL CUP

This caramel-hued, sweet-tasting brew was inspired by plants foraged on the coastal cliffs of St. Ives, Cornwall, in the southwest of England. We would suggest dunking in a Cornish Fairing cookie to provide a bonus ginger hit, but a gingersnap makes a good substitute. To get a bracing taste of the Atlantic, add a sprinkle of bladder wrack (if you dare).

Serve: 1 teaspoon per cup
2 parts dried nettle leaves
1 part dried meadowsweet flowers
2 parts dried gorse flowers

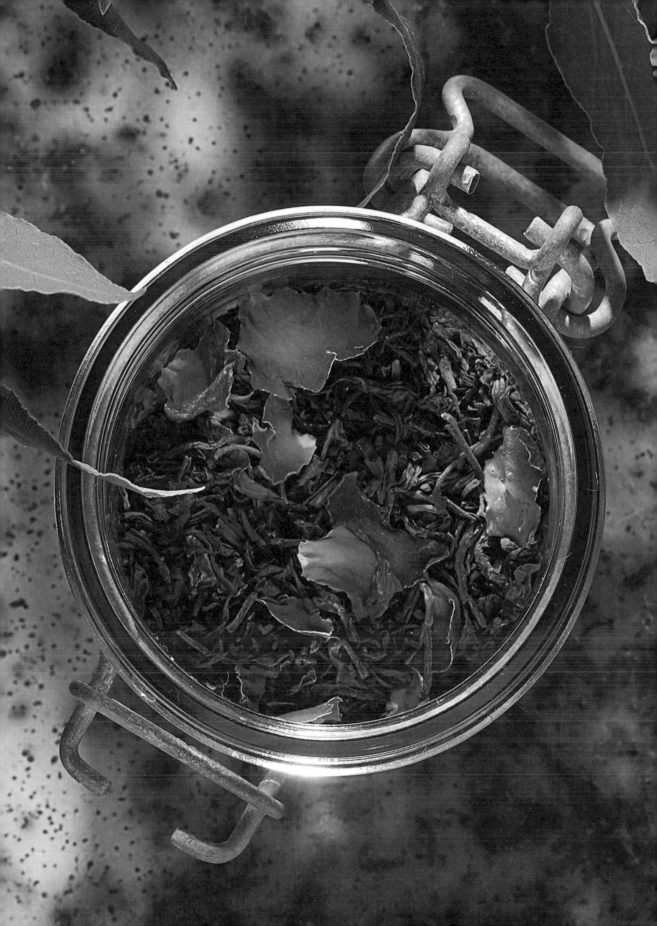

TEA TWISTS

These three blends are based on some of the most popular teas from around the world, each with a wild tea twist to make them an instant homemade success.

CHINA TEA WITH ROSE

Rose Congou tea (or China rose tea) is an ancient blend that is made by layering rose petals with tea leaves during their oxidization process. This allows for a floral fragrance to permeate the tea. For a shortcut version, you can simply mix dried rose petals with China black tea (you can, of course, use any black tea, but we think this works well with the mellow flavors of Keemum). Let rest for at least a couple of days to give the floral flavors time to infuse.

For a caffeine-free alternative, try substituting the black tea with another dried leaf; we've found the combination of rose and nettle is a winner.

Serve: 1 teaspoon per cup
2 parts China black tea
1 part dried rose petals

THRIFTY SHADES OF (EARL) GREY

The popular aromatic Earl Grey is black tea that has been flavored with bergamot oil. Anyone who grows bee balm (*Monarda didyma*) can take advantage of its bergamot-esque flavor and blend it with black tea for a cheap home-made version. It's not a totally accurate replica, but there are enough similar shades to make it an enjoyable alternative for Earl Grey fans.

Serve: 1 teaspoon per cup
2 parts black tea
1 part dried *Monarda didyma* leaves

Crush the dried *Monarda didyma* leaves, combine with the black tea, and give them a couple of days infusion time before using. Earl Grey itself is often combined with dried citrus peel and cornflower petals, so try using either to add a little color to your own blend.

QUICK MOROCCAN MINT TEA

A true Moroccan mint tea should be made precisely and with fresh mint (see page 137), but this dried version still tastes great and is well worth making in a big batch to keep in your dried tea collection.

Serve: 1 teaspoon per cup
3 parts green tea
2 parts dried mint leaves

Simply mix the green tea with crushed, dried mint leaves and use 1 teaspoon per cup. To increase authenticity, you can pile sugar into your cup, but we prefer it without. Moroccans are also known to add other ingredients to their mint teas, including lemon verbena, star anise, saffron, and wormwood,* so try experimenting with some of these flavors, too.

* Wormwood comes with a warning: it is intensely bitter, so only a touch is required.

DAY AND NIGHT

Imagine having the same meal for breakfast, lunch, and dinner. And imagine not changing that meal the next day, or the next—even if you wake feeling a little groggy or are eager to wind down for an early night. Just as we appreciate some timely order to our eating habits, we like to vary our tea drinking accordingly. Here, then, are three teas to see you safely through the day.

MORNING AFTER THE NIGHT BEFORE TEA

Everyone swears by their own hangover cure, but there has been little scientific research or indeed evidence to support their effectiveness. The hazardous nature of our job has led us to try most of them over the years, and we think this tea blend is as good as any. Borage and turmeric will help detoxify your polluted body, and peppermint will help ease your stomach and freshen your stale, beery breath.

Serve: 1 teaspoon per cup
1 part borage leaves (fresh or dried)
1 part turmeric
3 parts dried peppermint leaves

AFTER DINNER TEA

Over done it on the apple pie? Then this tea will aid digestion and improve your stomach's ills. In India, fennel seeds are eaten as an alternative to afterdinner mints, so mint and fennel make an obvious combination, and ginger is good at soothing upset stomachs and fighting indigestion. Together, their powerful flavor will also make you feel fresh and ready to face the rest of the day.

Serve: 2 teaspoons per cup
1 part dried mint leaves
1 part fennel seeds
1 part dried ginger pieces, or ground ginger

SUE'S "HOP TO BED" TEA

One of our go-to experts on the well-being benefits of natural ingredients is Sue Mullet, who uses her knowledge well by producing some amazing elixirs at Bath Botanical Gin Distillery and Herbal Apothecary. She also blends teas, with one of her most popular being this concoction, which is designed to be taken before heading off to bed. The hops, valerian, lavender, and linden flower all have calming properties that will set you in the right mood for sleep. We like it so much that we stole the recipe from under Sue's nose while she was taking a nap.

Serve: 1 teaspoon per cup
3 parts dried hops
1 part valerian roots
1 part dried linden flowers
1 part dried lavender flowers

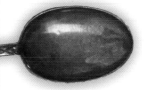

SPRING AND SUMMER BLENDS

Spring and summer see us working at our hardest in the yard—weeding and sowing, digging and hoeing, cutting and mowing—but mostly puffing and blowing (and cursing) trying to get the barbecue grill to work properly. These teas provide some light refreshment from the seasonal stresses and strains.

SUMMER FLOWER TEA

This blend combines some of our favorite floral ingredients, each readily available from our yards during the summer months. Elderflower and marigold are the more delicate constituents, so they each have double quantities; the chamomile adds a unique fruity fragrance and the hint of lavender provides a subtle, soothing summer tingle at the finish. For an alternative flower arrangement, you could try substituting the chamomile with rose petals.

Serve: 2 teaspoons per cup
2 parts dried elderflowers
2 parts dried marigolds
1 part dried lavender flowers
1 part dried chamomile flowers

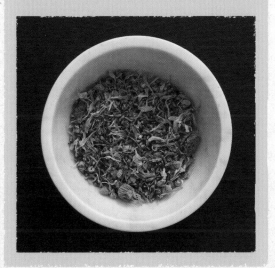

SPRING GREEN LEAF TEA

There is a time in spring, when the landscape is cloaked in every shade of green imaginable and garden growth goes into overdrive. For the first time in the year, we have to put in a hard stint of work to keep on top of things. This is a tea for such moments of hard work—an invigorating, leafy brew that refreshes the system like a drop of oil in a squeaky pair of secateurs. It's equally good served hot or ice cold with a slice of lemon.

Serve: 2 teaspoon per cup
2 parts dried lemon
  balm leaves
1 part dried mint leaves
2 parts dried blackberry
  leaves
1 part dried rosemary
  leaves

THE THIRSTY GARDENER'S TEA

For us, summer arrives when the first spruce and pine tips emerge, and ends when our community garden hops ripen. This tea is one of our most refreshing summer drinks, quenching our thirst and acting as a foil for spruce tips, hops, or other aromatic additions, such as rosemary, which can be freshly plucked and dunked into the brew. The hoppy recipe also provided the inspiration for our tea-flavored beer, expertly brewed by St Austell Brewery (see *page 150*).

Serve: 1 teaspoon per cup
1 part dried lemon
  verbena leaves
1 part green tea

Optional
2 fresh hops/5 spruce
  or pine tips/a sprig of
  rosemary

FALL AND WINTER BLENDS

Hot drinks come into their own during the colder months of the year and any winter chills can be banished further with the introduction of some warming spice. These blends are among the coziest brews you can find, providing some rich seasonal flavors that will help defend you against the elements.

SPICED ORANGE HOT CHOCOLATE MIX

There are times during long, dark evenings when the comfort of warming spice isn't enough and the extra satisfaction of indulgence is required. Time to crack open the cocoa. This blend will bring extra cheer to your hot chocolate with its tickling of orange and spice.

Blend	Hot chocolate
1 part dried orange peel	1⅓ cups of milk
1 part cinnamon stick, crumbled	2 tablespoons unsweetened cocoa powder
1 part dried ginger pieces or ground ginger	2 teaspoons spiced orange hot chocolate mix
1 part dried bay leaf	2 teaspoons sugar

To make, simply add 1⅓ cups of milk to a saucepan (the extra is to allow for evaporation) and steadily bring to a boil. Take the milk off the heat and whisk in the cocoa powder, then add the spices and sugar. Return to the heat and gently simmer for 5–10 minutes, stirring as you go. Strain and serve.

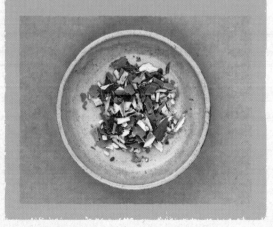

HARVEST BREW

Fall is a busy time for wild tea makers— digging roots from the garden, plucking fruit from trees, and roaming the thickets for forage-worthy goods—and this ruddy brew is a reward for those harvesting efforts.

Serve: 2 teaspoons per cup
2 parts dried apple
1 part dried beet
1 part dried rose hips
1 part dried ginger pieces or ground ginger

Chop or grind the sweet apple, earthy beet, fruity rose hips, and spicy ginger. Combine and steep in a cup of hot water for at least 5 minutes before basking in a healthy harvest glow.

A FESTIVE BREW

If you're a fan of the festive flavors that go into a mulled wine, but want something free from booze, then this is the brew for you.

Serve: 2 teaspoons per cup
3 parts dried black currant leaves
3 parts dried hibiscus flowers
2 parts dried rose hips
2 parts cinnamon stick, crumbled
1 part licorice root
1 part dried ginger pieces or ground ginger

Blend the ingredients and steep for 10 minutes in a cup of boiling water, then breathe in its heady aroma and sip. On its own it makes a soothing tea, but for an extra kick, try adding a pinch of chili powder to each cup.

HEALTHY BREWS

Although some of the health claims surrounding our tea ingredients are wilder than the back of Rich's community garen, there is evidence that many of them can do some good. These teas have been created with their health and well-being properties in mind.

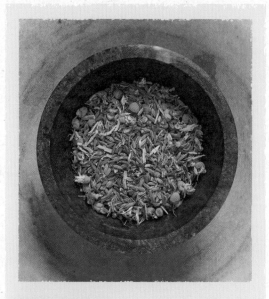

COLD-BUSTING TEA

It may be true that there's no cure for the common cold, but you can certainly perk yourself up with a healthy dose of vitamins. These ingredients provide an alphabet soup of vitamin goodness, with C common to them all.

Serve: 3 teaspoons per cup
2 parts dried rose hips
2 parts dried elderberries
2 parts dried echinacea leaves
1 part dried lemon peel

Steep for 10 minutes (or simmer in water to extract even more flavor) in a cup of hot water and sip slowly when the cold bug is next doing the rounds.

NEW MOM'S (AND OLD DAD'S) TEA

One of the biggest boom areas for healthy teas is blends designed for new moms. Nettle and fennel are often a feature of these concoctions because they can aid the production of breast milk, while a pinch of chamomile can help to keep mom calm during times of tiny tantrums. Seeing as we're a couple of old dads, we cannot vouch for this tea's effectiveness, but drink it anyway because it tastes great.

Serve: 2 teaspoons per cup
2 parts dried nettle leaves
2 parts fennel seeds
1 part dried chamomile flowers

ENERGY TEA

Can a cup of tea really give you energy? If any tea can, then it's this one. It combines the eye-widening stimulants of yerba mate with the all-round goodness of licorice, and an equal measure of mint for some extra flavor.

Serve: 2 teaspoons per cup
1 part dried yerba mate leaves
1 part licorice root
1 part dried mint leaves

Steep in a cup of hot water for at least 5 minutes before drinking— it may not give you enough energy to run a marathon, but it will certainly snap you out of a work-time slumber.

CHAI

There is an infinite array of masala chais you could make, but there are essentially two ways to make them: with care, love and fresh ingredients (see *page 138*) or with pre-made, dried blends for people with less time on their hands (read on).

USING THE BLENDS

For each of these blends, you'll need 1 tablespoon per cup and you can make them with milk, water, or a combination of both. For speedy chais, simply steep the ingredients in just-boiled liquid for at least 5 minutes; for a fuller flavor, simmer them in a saucepan for 10 minutes. Sweeten to taste.

BASIC GINGER CHAI

If you take a survey of the five key ingredients for masala chai, this selection might come out on top. It's certainly a good place to start before experimenting with your own blends. We like a touch of black pepper for an extra kick, but add no more than a quarter part per batch or a pinch per cup.

Serve: 1 tablespoon per cup
3 parts black tea
2 parts dried ginger pieces or ground ginger
2 parts green cardamom pods
1 part cinnamon stick
1 part fennel seeds

Chop, grind, or mash all the ingredients before mixing. Add a grind of pepper if you want a fiery kick.

NICK'S ROSE GARDEN CHAI

For this chai, Nick has delved into the yard for three ingredients to infuse with the more exotic spices. Rose petals add fragrance to complement the cardamom; fennel seeds give the tea some earthy, aniselike depth; and the spicy ginger has been dropped in place of the softer spice of bay leaf.

Serve: 1 tablespoon per cup
3 parts black tea
1 part dried rose petals
1 part cinnamon stick, crumbled
1 part fennel seeds
2 parts dried bay leaves
2 parts cardamom pods

RICH'S CHILI CHOCCY CHAI

If he was being honest, Rich came up with the name before the recipe but, luckily, this blend turned out to be a winner. It's a fine chai to sip on winter evenings—the chili will warm you up while the chocolate addition adds a luxurious texture.

Serve: 1 tablespoon per cup
3 parts black tea
2 parts green cardamom pods
1 part cinnamon stick, crumbled
½ part dried chili pepper
1 part dried ginger pieces or ground ginger
2 parts good-quality semisweet chocolate, chopped

Combine all the ingredients apart from the chocolate, which you should add to each cup before serving. Serve it with a swirl of cream and be a super-chai guy.

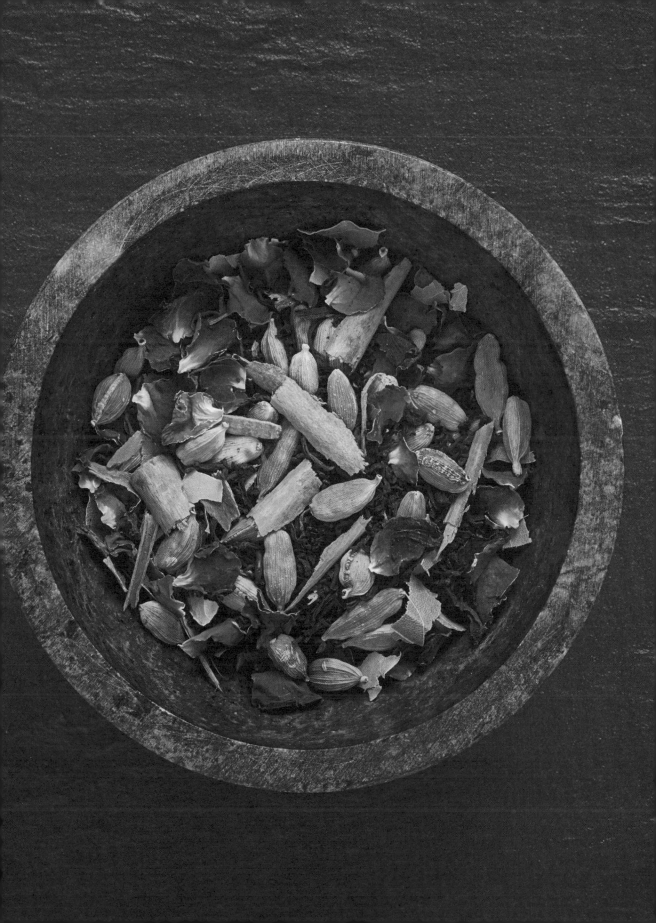

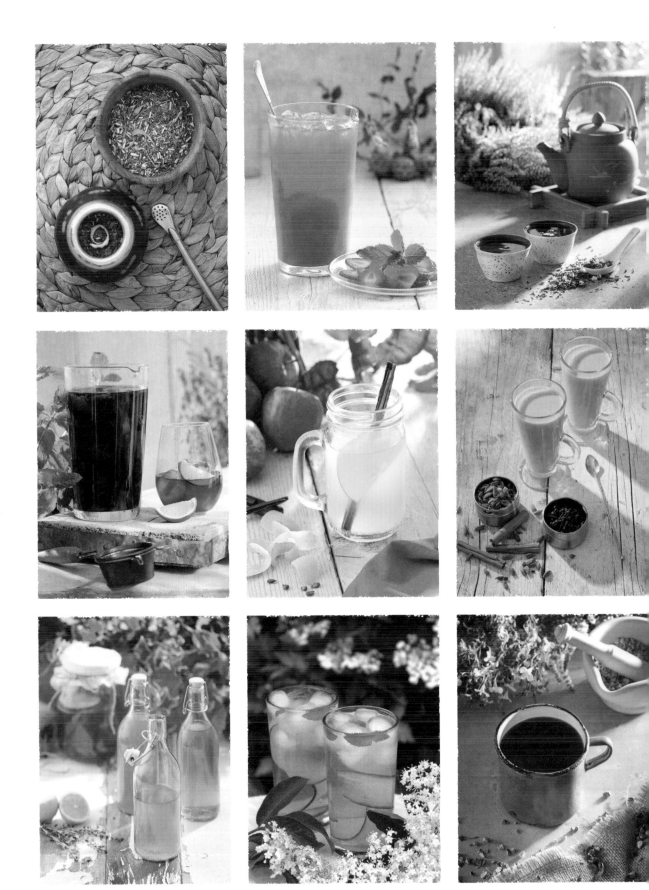

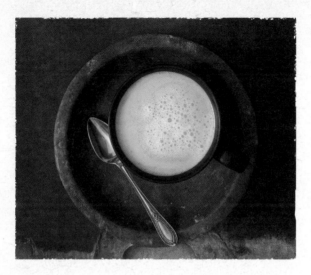

Special Teas, Coffees, and Other Concoctions

In this section we feature some of our favorite special brews that take a little more effort than simply dunking an ingredient in hot water. We've been fermenting, roasting, cooling and mixing to produce some amazing drinks from around the world, each of them easy to make in your own home. So clear some space in the kitchen and let's brew.

Yerba Mate

Yerba mate is a smoky-tasting, antioxidant-packed brew made from the stems and leaves of *Ilex paraguariensis*, a species of holly native to the subtropical rain forests of Argentina, Brazil, and Paraguay. The beverage was first imbibed by the indigenous Guaraní and Tupi communities, with its popularity spreading across the continent through the teachings of traveling Jesuit missionaries. More recently, the drink was brought to the attention of a worldwide audience of armchair dwellers during the 2018 FIFA World Cup, when many of the South American soccer-playing stars could be seen disembarking their team buses clutching distinctive yerba mate gourds. Sipping yerba mate in social groups is common practice in South America. To make like a pro, grab a gourd, load it with leaves, and share with your yerba mate pals.

GROW IT

Ilex paraguariensis' penchant for subtropical climes confines it to South America, where this broadleaf, evergreen shrub can grow to heights of 50 feet. In order to prepare it for tea-making purposes, the leaves and stems are cut from the mature plant and are heated to halt the oxidization process. The plant parts are then dried and stored for up to a year to help intensify flavors before heading gourd-ward and made into tea.

DRINK IT

You can make your yerba mate in a mug, but the delivery system of choice is the calabash gourd paired with a bombilla—a stainless steel straw with a perforated basket at its end to prevent the leaves from entering your mouth and ruining your herbal hit. The gourd is filled halfway with leaves before adding hot (not boiling) water. Yerba mate doesn't stew like a traditional black leaf tea, so the drinking vessel can be topped with water regularly with the leaves left to infuse several times before discarding.

MIX IT

Utilize the smoky flavors of yerba mate to make some magical mixes of your own.

Minty Yerba Mate

Combine dried garden mint with equal measures of yerba mate for a minty mix that smells a little like menthol cigarettes (but is considerably healthier to consume).

Yerba Mate Buoy

A smoky, seaside-inspired combination. Make a mix of 2 parts yerba mate, 1 part gorse, 1 part chopped, dried rose hips, and a tiny sprinkle of dried seaweed.

Jolly Holly

Step into Christmas with this festive fireside blend: 2 parts yerba mate, 1 part ginger, a curl of dried orange peel, and a dash of cinnamon.

For a yerba mate energy tea packed with pick-me-up-ability, turn to *page 129*.

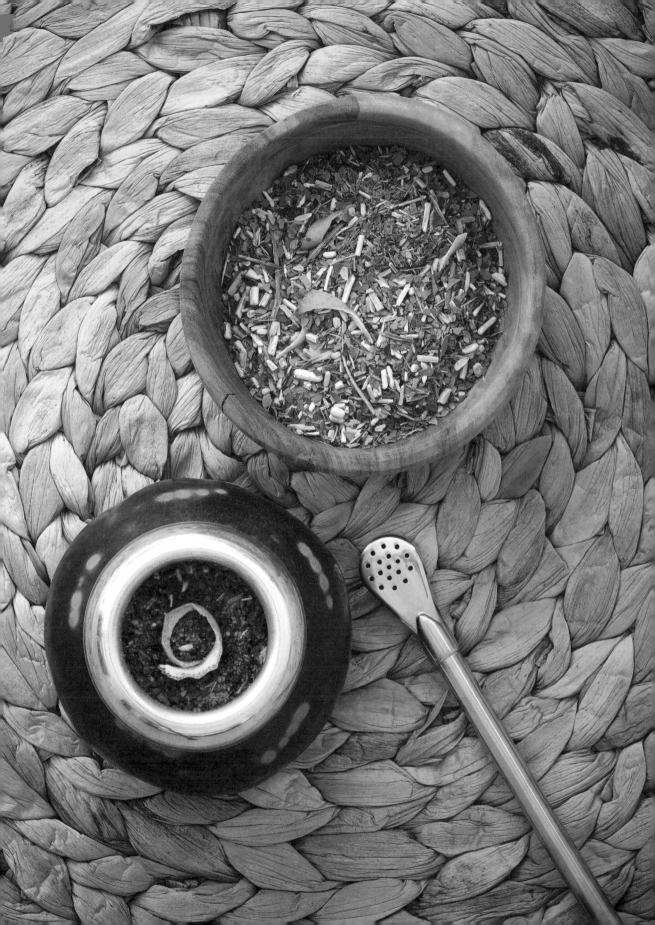

GROW YOUR OWN YERBA CUP

Yerba mate is traditionally served in a hollowed-out calabash (*Lagenaria siceraria*), also known as the bird house or bottle gourd. The calabash grows best in warm climates, but we've had success growing ours here in the UK in a sheltered, south-facing garden.

HOW TO GROW

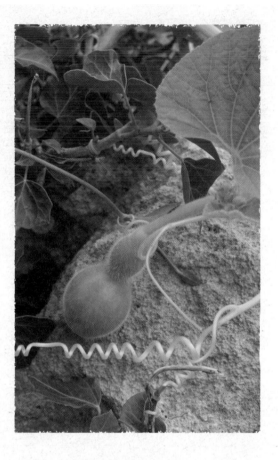

1 Sow the seed indoors from March onward into individual containers. Push the seed, edge side down, to prevent rot, then cover with a layer of vermiculite or potting mix.

2 Calabash, like most cucurbits, outgrow their pots quickly, so plant them into larger plant pots before they become root bound.

3 Move your calabashes into a cold frame or the open ground from April onward. Calabashes are best grown on a sunny site, in a rich soil that has had plenty of organic matter added. If you have the time and inclination, prep your preferred site before planting.

4 Calabashes love to climb—the plant will shoot out tendrils that will latch onto anything for support—so grow them up and over a trellis to allow the fruit to dangle freely. Allowing them to ramble across the ground is fine, too, but calabashes resting on the ground tend to grow misshapen and you may lose that glorious bowling pin profile.

5 Water regularly throughout the season. Poking a stake into the soil where the taproot lies will help you to water where the plant needs it the most. Better still, cut the bottom off a plastic bottle and slide it— neck end first—through the stake. Push the neck into the soil and use it as a funnel for maximum watering efficiency.

HOW TO DRY

When completely mature, chop the gourd from its stem and let sit somewhere cool that has good air circulation. The drying process will take a few months, so be patient. Once dry, lop off the top, where the neck begins to widen into the bottom. Lightly sand it with a fine-grade sandpaper and coat the outer skin with a layer or two of varnish to protect your new drinking vessel from yerba mate spillage.

Moroccan Mint Tea

Adding a handful of leaves to a mug of boiling water makes an excellent mint tea, but for maximum minty pleasures, make like a Moroccan. It's a ritualistic process and everyone who makes it has their own theory on how it should be done. This is the version Nick stole from a French tea maker, Mario, at a riad in Marrakesh, who claimed it was by far the best method—and we have no reason to doubt him.

Makes: 1 teapot
2 tablespoons green tea
1 large handful of
   fresh mint leaves
2 tablespoons sugar

MORE THAN MINT

Although mint is the most popular, Moroccans use a variety of herbs in their teas. Experiment with variations of this recipe, using sage, lemon balm, lemon verbena, or whatever else appeals to you.

1 First rinse out and warm the teapot with some boiling water.

2 Put the green tea into the pot. Ideally, you want dried loose leaves (Moroccans prefer a version called Chinese gunpowder green tea) but you can get away with a few tea bags if you're desperate (meaning you can probably skip the next two steps—just don't tell Mario).

3 Fill a heatproof glass with boiling water, pour it onto the tea, and let stand for about a minute before gently swishing the teapot and pouring the infused liquid back into the glass. This is good stuff known as "the soul of the tea."

4 Now you need to wash the green tea that's left in the teapot to get rid of some bad stuff (bitter flavors). Pour another glass of boiling water into the teapot, let it stand for a 2–3 minutes, swish, then pour the liquid away.

5 Grab a large handful of fresh mint (or two if you have tiny hands) and stuff it into the teapot along with the "soul of the tea" from step 3 and the sugar. While 2 tablespoons is a lot of sugar by our standards, many Moroccans will add more than three times that amount, so feel free to adjust to your own personal tastes. Tea bag cheats should add their green tea now.

6 If you have a teapot that is heated on the stove, you can fill it with water and bring it to a gentle boil before serving. Alternatively, fill it to the brim with freshly boiled water.

7 At this point, we would usually reach for a spoon and stir the tea, but if you want to impress your pals with your tea-making abilities, stir it the traditional way by pouring out a glass and immediately pouring it back into the teapot. Mario repeated this five times.

8 At long last, your tea is now ready to serve. For a final flourish of frothy authenticity, hold the spout high above the glass and pour.

Masala Chai

Masala Chai is the spiced tea that is served everywhere from chaiwala stalls on bustling Indian roadsides to restaurants, bars, and cafés throughout the world. This is a basic recipe that centers on the essential ingredient of all good masala chais: cardamom. Add a few complementary spices to the fragrant green pods and simmer yourself a simple spicy treat.

Makes: 1 large mug
4 green cardamom pods
½ cinnamon stick
 (2 inches in length)
2 cloves
1 cup water
1 cup milk
2 teaspoons (or 2 tea
 bags) black tea
Sugar, to taste

1 Gently mash the cardamom pods using a mortar and pestle until they are cracked and bruised, then put them into a saucepan with the cinnamon, cloves, and water.

2 Bring to a boil, then turn the heat down, fit a lid on the pan, and gently simmer for 10 minutes.

3 Add the milk and bring the liquid back to a boil, stirring constantly. When it reaches boiling point, take it off the heat, add the tea, put the lid back on, and let it infuse for about 4 minutes.

4 Strain into cups* and serve, sweetening to taste.

* *Traditionally, Indians use small glasses known as "cutting chai"—the smaller portion "cutting the chai in half."*

Variations:
If you want even more spice in your chai, try adding a few extra ingredients, such as some grated ginger, a bay leaf, a peppercorn or two, or a few fennel seeds.

BLACK TEA CHOICE

We think masala chai works best with a robust black tea—Assam being our preference. This recipe makes a fairly mild and milky chai, so you can easily add another 1–2 teaspoons of tea if you want something stronger.

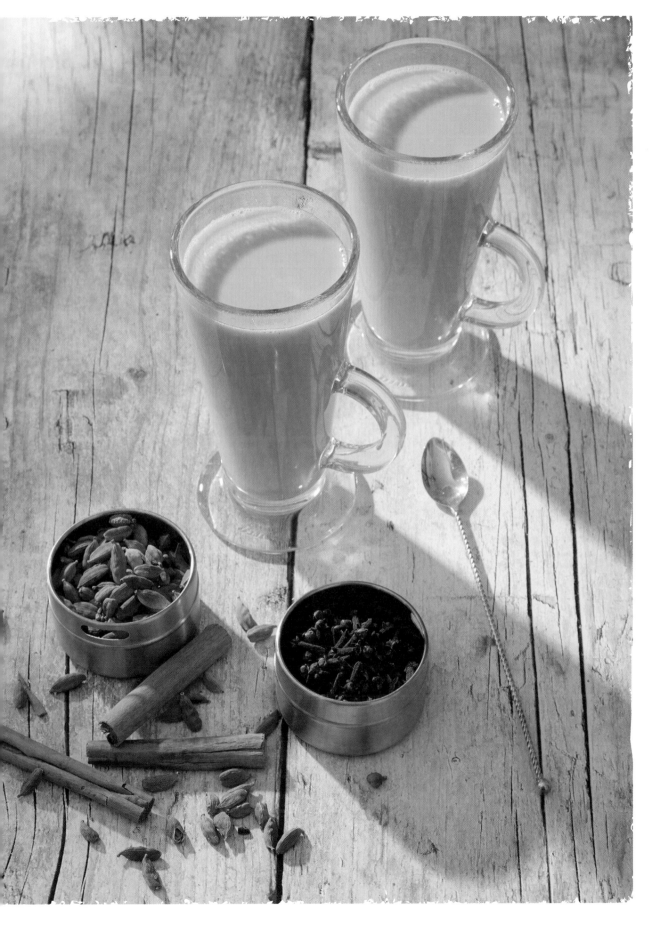

Genmaicha

Genmaicha is a Japanese blend of green tea and toasted rice that has turned out to be one of our favorite brews. There is a theory that the rice was originally added to bulk out the green tea and make it a cheaper drink, but our Japanese tea correspondent* suggests it was developed as a way of adding a good aroma to any green teas lacking in the olfactory department. The tea is also called "popcorn tea," because some of the grains are prone to popping (like popcorn), providing the potential for some kitchen amusement to anyone making it.

Makes: 1 cup
½ cup white rice
½ cup green tea

* *Nagahiro Yasumori of Horaido Tea Shop. It was Master Horaido who first came up with the idea for the blend in the 1920s.*

** *The Japanese also blend unbrowned white rice with tea, but they use it more sparingly, because when they look in the pot, the white rice reminds them of the tea plant's flowers, and a good tea plantation has few flowers.*

*** *You will have to listen for a lack of bubbling water to know if it has dried out. Or use a transparent lid.*

Although *genmai* means "brown rice," it's white rice you'll need for this recipe—the roasting turns it brown.** We've had success with basmati and long-grain rice but, for authenticity, use a Japanese-style glutinous rice (often referred to as sushi rice).

1 Before roasting, you need to steam or boil the rice, and before that you have to remove as much starch as possible so the grains don't stick together (which is a particular curse with glutinous rice). Soak in cold water for 10 minutes, then rinse until the water runs clear.

2 Next, boil or steam your rice. If you have a preferred method, use it; otherwise, put the rice into a saucepan with the same volume of water plus a third. Put the lid on and slowly bring to a boil. Turn down the heat and simmer for 10–15 minutes (or until there is no water left). Turn off the heat and let stand for 10 minutes. Resist the temptation to lift the lid throughout.***

3 When cooked, shake the rice in a drainer to remove excess water and spread the grains on a plate to cool and dry. If they're still sticking together, shaking them in the strainer when dried should separate them. Spread them out on a nonstick baking sheet or one lined with parchment paper and roast them in a preheated oven at 400°F for about 25 minutes, until golden brown.

4 Let the rice cool, then combine with the green tea at a 50/50 ratio and use 1 teaspoon per serving. This tea is best brewed at a temperature slightly below boiling point, so take the water off the heat right before it boils or let the water stand for a few minutes before pouring.

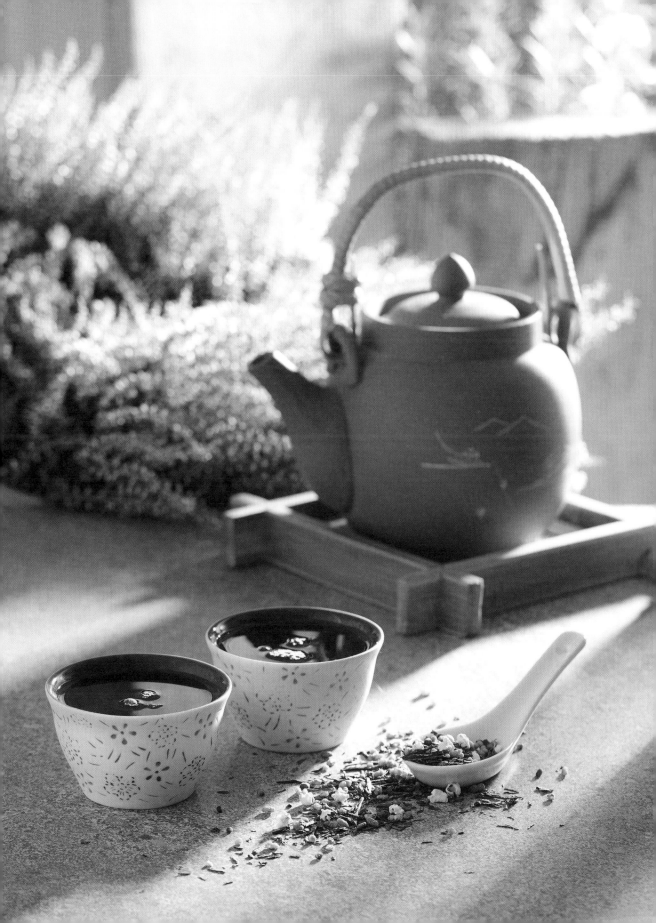

Turmeric Latte

Turmeric latte, often referred to as "golden milk," has grown in popularity over the last few years, initially migrating from Asian kitchens to trendy cafés before becoming a relatively common sight on beverage menus in all types of establishments. As with all fashionable recipes, everyone will have their own theory on how best to make it; ours is based on simplicity. Whisk one up first thing in the morning or last thing at night and bask in its soothing golden glow.

Makes: 1 cup
1¼ cups of milk
1 teaspoon freshly grated (or 1 teaspoon ground) turmeric
½ teaspoon freshly grated (or 5 teaspoons ground) ginger
¼ teaspoon cinnamon
Honey or maple syrup, to taste

1 If you have fresh turmeric and ginger roots, grate them finely into a small saucepan, otherwise ground powder is fine. Add the cinnamon—either crumbled from a stick or already ground.

2 Pour the milk into the pan—you can be lazy and use your mug to measure it instead of a measuring cup, but measure out an extra quarter of the mug to allow for evaporation. This is a great recipe for trying out milk alternatives, with coconut milk and almond milk being our favorites.

3 Slowly heat the mixture, occasionally whisking it gently to disperse the spices. Turn off the heat just before it boils and give a quick final whisk, putting a little more vigor into it than during the earlier stages; this will give your latte a pleasantly frothy texture.

4 Pour the latte into your cup (straining it if you've used fresh ingredients) and sweeten it with honey or maple syrup to your desired taste. If you want to add an extra visual flourish, sprinkle some cinnamon over the surface.

PEPPER POWER

Some people add a pinch of black pepper to their lattes to make them healthier. Turmeric contains curcumin (responsible for its color), which is claimed by some people to be an antioxidant and antibacterial, but our bodies aren't good at absorbing it. Piperine, which is found in pepper, is said to aid curcumin's absorption; and thankfully, pepper's spicy notes won't ruin your golden milk.

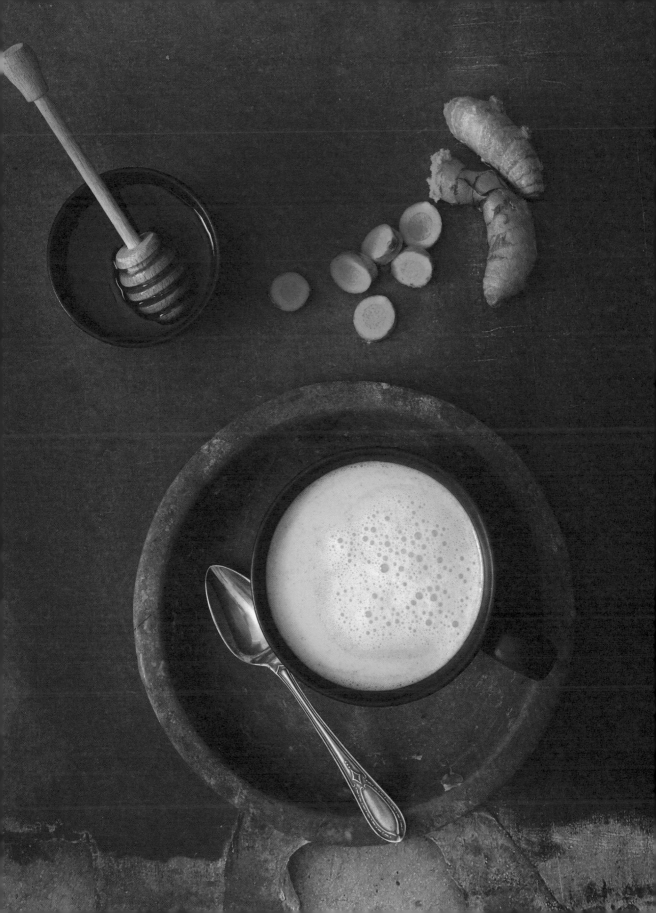

Roasted Barley Tea

Barley isn't the most obvious crop to grow on a small scale, but the patch in his garden that Rich reserves for cereals produces enough to make a few bottles of beer and several pots of this tea. It's a popular beverage in Korea, where it's known as *boricha* and is served hot or cold. We've never visited Korea so can't compare it to our locally brewed cup, but our attempts have produced a pleasing nutty, toasty drink that's a little like beer but without the booze.

Makes: 1 cup
3 tablespoons barley
1⅔ cups water
1–2 teaspoons honey,
    to taste

1 You can buy preroasted barley or you can use regular barley and roast it yourself—we've found pearled barley works the best. To create the desired roastiness, either heat it in a heavy saucepan or skillet over medium heat for 5–10 minutes, regularly tossing and turning the grains, or lay out on a baking sheet and put in a preheated oven at 400°F and bake for about 15 minutes. They're ready when they take on a deep golden color (too much roasting will unleash a less-appealing burned flavor).

2 To make the tea, put the roasted barley into a saucepan and fill with water.

3 Bring the water to a boil, then cover with a lid and simmer over low heat. We find 15 minutes is enough, however, simmer it for longer for a more intensely flavored drink or just 10 minutes for a lighter brew.

4 If you have a sweet tooth, add 1–2 teaspoons of honey, which perfectly complements the nutty goodness of this beverage.

5 Strain the liquid into a mug and serve hot, or chill it for a cold caffeine-free alternative to iced coffee.

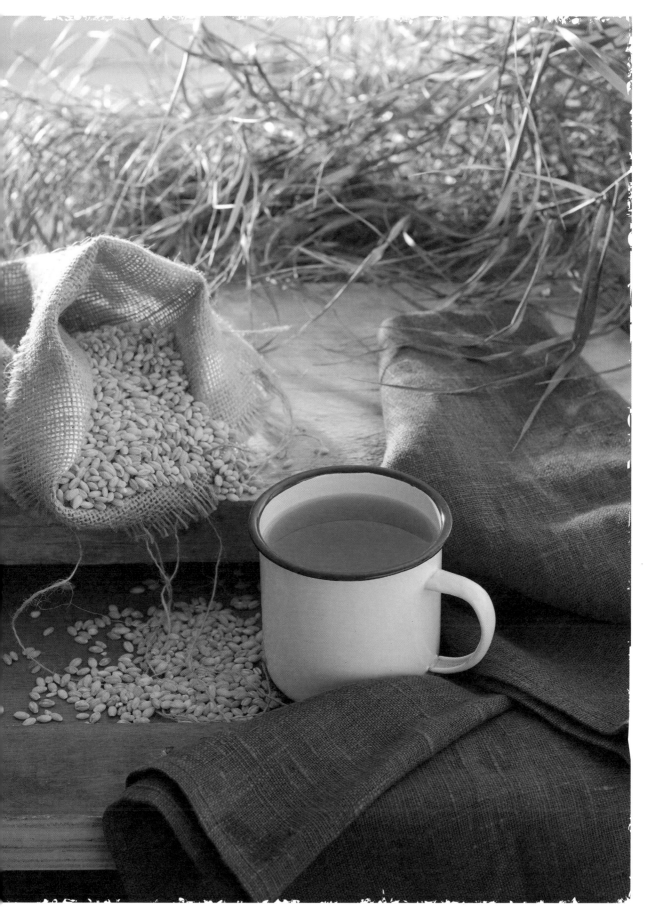

Sun Teas

Sun teas are one of summer's treats and involve slowly infusing the flavors of your chosen ingredients into water by using only the power of the sun. It's a simple, fuss-free process. Just put your ingredients into a pitcher, fill with water, and set aside in a sunny spot. Within a few hours, you'll have a flavorsome drink that can be enjoyed straight from the pitcher or chilled in the refrigerator.

This slow method of brewing rewards you with drinks that have slightly different characteristics to teas that use boiling water, with lighter, cleaner, and fresher flavors. Start them in the morning and they'll be ready for lunch, making a great feature of a shared meal with friends. You can even top off the pitcher with more water as you drink it. Over the next four pages, we've got three of our favorite sun tea recipes, but part of the fun in making them is strolling around the yard and filling a pitcher with whatever you want—so let the summer sun send your imagination wild.

A SIMPLE LEMON SUN TEA

This sun tea is as basic as it gets and lets you appreciate the flavors of a slow, low-temperature tea infusion with just enough lemon to give it some citrusy freshness.

Makes: 5 cups
4 black tea bags
½ a lemon
5 cups cold water

1 Put the tea bags into a pitcher with the lemon (squeeze the juice into the pitcher before adding the rind). Fill with cold water and cover. If your pitcher doesn't have a fitted lid, use a clean dish towel, plastic wrap, or an alternative makeshift cover, such as a plate.

2 Let infuse for 2–3 hours before serving immediately, or chill in the refrigerator for later.

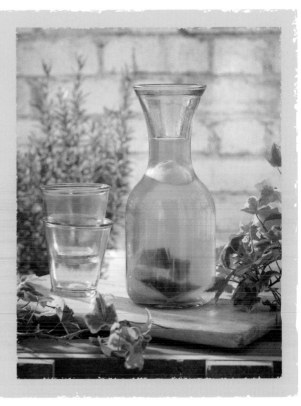

PEACH AND RASPBERRY SUN TEA

If it's a good year for raspberries, there are times when we can't pick them fast enough, so a sun tea is great for a quick pick-and-brew on the more bountiful days. Tart raspberries love joining forces with sweet juicy peaches, and they both work well in the presence of black tea, which makes this recipe one of our fruitiest favorites.

Makes: 5 cups
4 black tea bags
2 peaches, sliced
1 large handful of raspberries
2 slices of lemon
5 cups cold water

1 We don't grow peaches, but we choose the ripest and juiciest specimens available, because nothing short of perfectly ripe will do for this brew. When satisfied with your peachy haul, wash, slice, and add them to a pitcher.

2 You also need ripe raspberries—after thoroughly rinsing them, throw them into the pitcher whole. Add the black tea bags, slices of lemon, and top off with cold water.

3 Cover the pitcher and set aside to infuse for 2–3 hours before drinking or refrigerating for later. This recipe benefits from stirring well before serving, so grab a long-handle spoon and rattle it around the liquid with some determination. Strain into glasses and serve with ice and a slice of lemon.

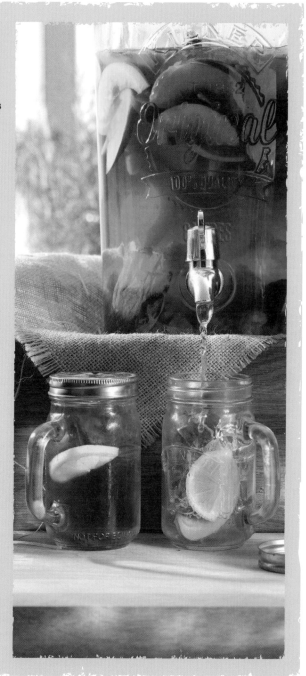

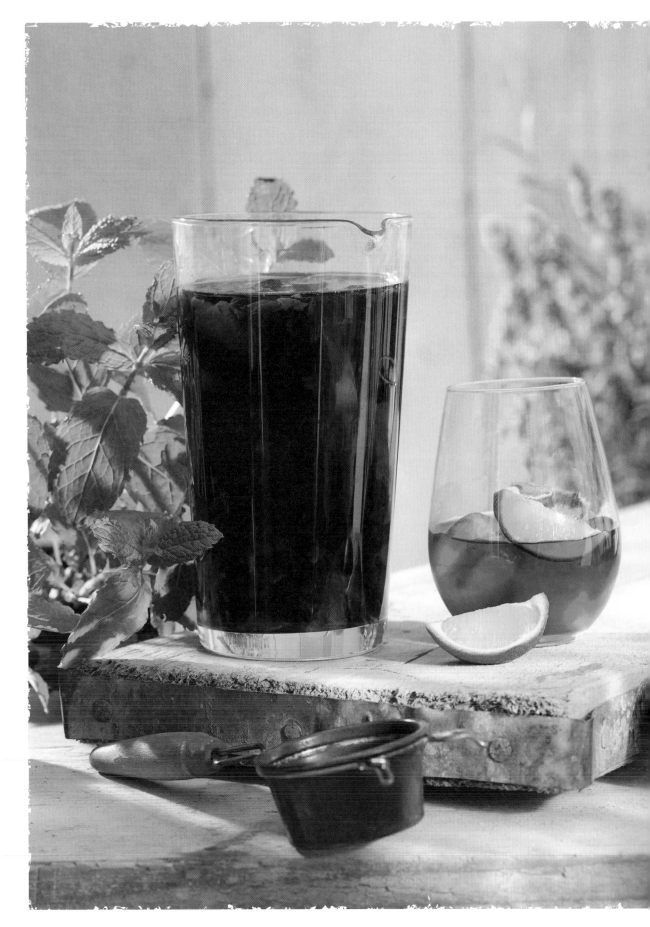

TROPICAL HIBISCUS SUN TEA

Hibiscus flowers could be made specifically for sun teas. Not only do their tart, fruity flavors make perfect summer sipping, but you also get the added visual bonus of the tea steadily reddening over time until it reaches a deep crimson hue. In this caffeine-free recipe, we've ramped up the tartness a notch with lime—some fruits are reluctant to release their full flavor in an infusion, but just a small amount of lime juice will add a lip-smacking sourness to this tropically refreshing mix.

Makes: 5 cups
2 handfuls of dried hibiscus flowers
1 handful of fresh mint leaves
¼ of a lime
1 thumb-size lump of ginger
5 cups cold water

1 Drop the dried hibiscus flowers into a pitcher. Grab the fresh mint leaves, crush, and tear them a little to start releasing their minty oils, then add them to the pitcher.

2 Squeeze the lime juice into the pitcher.* Follow it with the juiceless chunk of rind.

3 Coarsely chop the ginger and bruise it to help release its sweet spicy flavors—a pestle or the blunt end of a heavy knife are suitable implements. Drop these pieces into the pitcher and add the cold water.

4 Cover the pitcher and set aside to infuse for 2–3 hours before drinking or refrigerating for later. Strain into glasses and, if you're the kind who likes a garnish, you can add a sprig of mint or slice of lime.

A NOTE ON QUANTITIES

It's not worth getting too hung up on precise quantities for sun teas. The pitchers we use tend to be around 5-cup capacity, so our quantities will suit this volume, give or take a splash or two. You can also make single cup sun teas by filling smaller jars with a fraction of the ingredients.

ARE SUN TEAS SAFE?

Search for sun teas on the Internet and it won't be long before you'll find an article questioning their safety—this is because the sun can heat your mix to a temperature that encourages bacteria growth from tap water and foodstuffs that would otherwise be killed off by boiling water. To minimize risk, you can use purified water and make sure the ingredients are thoroughly clean before using them, infuse for no more than 3 hours in a cooler location, and put the resulting tea in the refrigerator if you won't be drinking it immediately. If you're the extremely cautious type, then "cold brew" instead—fill the pitcher with all the ingredients and infuse overnight in the refrigerator.

* *If you like extra-sour drinks, by all means add another quarter or two to the mix.*

SWEETENING YOUR SUN TEA

We tend not to sweeten sun teas, but if you need your hit of sugar, then you're better off adding it in liquid form so it can dissolve into the blend. Honey or a syrup should work well.

Boozy Teas

Tea isn't a drink to be simply enjoyed in its own right, it also makes a useful ingredient for numerous other beverages, especially alcoholic drinks.

BEER AND TEA: A WINNING COMBINATION

Tea and beer may seem like an unusual combination, but tea from the *Camellia sinensis* plant has a lot in common with hops—it provides flavor, aroma, and bitterness—so perhaps it's not so surprising that various types of teas have been included in beer recipes. Similarly, many of our wild tea ingredients have found their way into beery brews, so we figured one of our favorite blends, The Thirsty Gardener's Tea (see *page 127*), might make a decent beer.

In order to test this theory, we hopped down to Cornwall to meet brewing manager Rob Orton at the world renowned St Austell Brewery, who helped us make a beer for real. To work out which hop cultivars would work best with the lemon verbena and green tea, and to work out what quantity of each to use, our first task was to brew up a tea with those key flavoring ingredients—a common practice among brewers when conjuring up any new recipe.

But brewers get to enjoy another hot beverage before the hops and other flavoring ingredients are added. When malted barley is first mashed to extract the sugar and flavor from the grains, a small amount is poured out to gauge its sugar content. This hot, sweet liquid is similar to other malted barley drinks and is known as "brewer's breakfast," with the lucky brewers getting a mugful to see them through the morning.

The final tea-making duties occur once the beer is completely fermented. If it's felt that the beer needs a flavor boost, then another tea is made from the same ingredients used in the brewing process, and it is added to the cask during conditioning. If our results are anything to go by, tea and beer are indeed a winning combination.

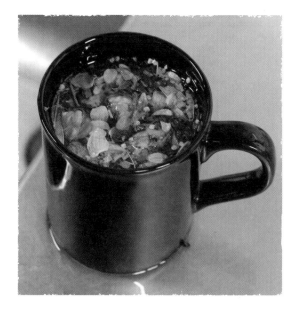

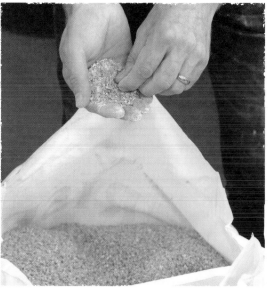

COCKTAILS

These days the fashion for fancy cocktails has resulted in bartenders using all kinds of ingredients to help create their own unique recipes, and teas are becoming one of the most popular additions around. However, using tea in boozy mixes isn't new. A drink known as gunfire, which consists of a simple combination of rum and black tea, has been enjoyed by the British Army since the nineteenth century, and hot toddies have long been made with black tea (see our recipe below).

You can also have fun inventing cocktails with one of your own wild teas—perhaps a mint tea mojito; an elderflower iced tea combined with the botanical flavors of gin; or even a dandelion coffee in an espresso martini.

And it's not just cocktails that have been enhanced with a drop or two of tea—tea can also be fermented to make a sparkling soda, kombucha (see *page 160*), or even wine.*

If you think of tea as simply another flavoring ingredient, there are unlimited options for making a wild and wonderful boozy brew.

OUR HOT TEA TODDY

This winter warmer will banish any sign of the sniffles.

Makes: 2 cups
2 cups water
2 teaspoons lemon juice
2 cloves
1 cinnamon stick (about 4 inches in length)
1 star anise, lightly crushed
¾-inch piece of ginger, peeled and coarsely chopped
2 tablespoons honey
1 teaspoon black tea (or 1 tea bag)
3 tablespoons brandy

1 Put the water, lemon juice, and spices into a saucepan and warm gently over low heat.

2 After a couple of minutes, add the honey and stir until dissolved.

3 Continue heating, stirring occasionally, for 10 minutes. Turn off the heat, add the tea and brandy, and let infuse for 2 minutes, stirring the mixture one or two times to tease out more flavor.

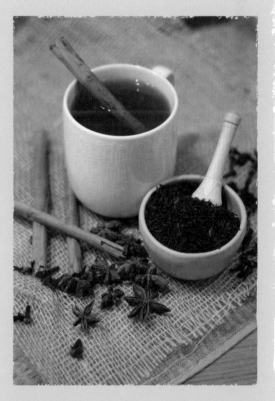

4 Remove from the heat and pour through a strainer into heat-resistant glasses or mugs.

* *Makers of country wines (elderflower wine, parsnip wine, and so on), often put black or green tea into their mix to give the resulting booze the kind of tannic crispness you would normally get from grape skins.*

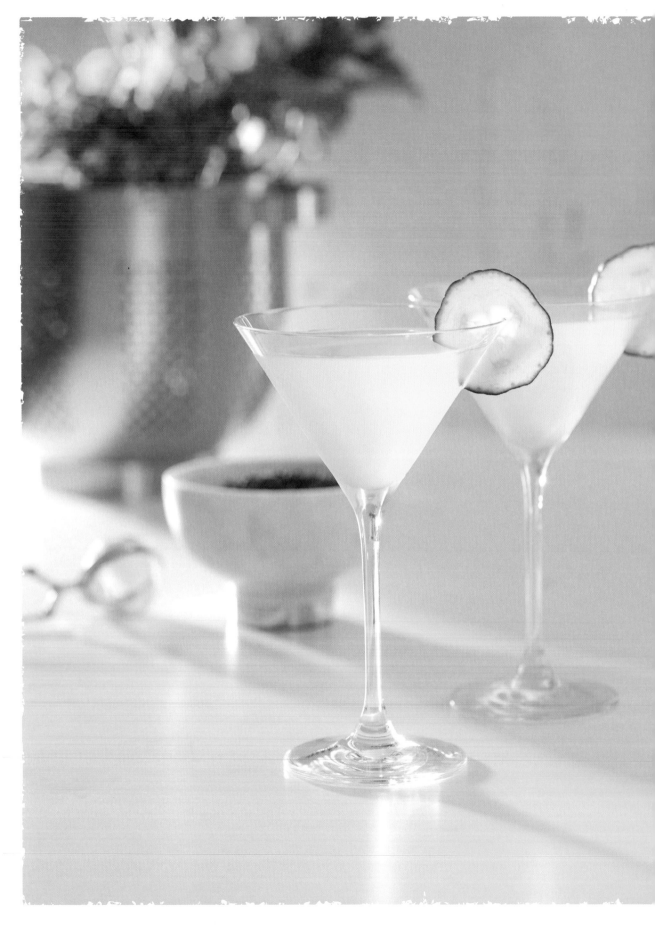

GREEN TEA AND CUCUMBER MARTINI*

You can make a simple wild tea martini by combining any flavored liquor (see below) with vermouth. We suggest starting out with this simple and refreshing green tea and cucumber infusion.

For the green tea and cucumber vodka
1 cup (8 oz) vodka or gin
2 teaspoons green tea
2-inch-long piece of cucumber

For the martini
¼ cup (2 oz) infused vodka or gin
1 tablespoon (½ oz) vermouth
Ice
Cucumber slices, to garnish

1 You can use gin or vodka for this infusion, but make sure it's a decent one and, if you've opted for gin, use one that hasn't been flavored by other dominant ingredients. The classic martini uses dry vermouth, but we think this recipe also lends itself to a sweet vermouth.

2 To flavor your liquor of choice, slice or chop the cucumber into small cubes and add to a lidded jar with the vodka and green tea.

3 Seal the lid, shake it vigorously, and set aside for 20 minutes. Strain the liquid into a separate jar or bottle.

4 To make the martini, first fill a cocktail shaker with crushed ice. Add the infused vodka and vermouth. Stir for 30 seconds (or shake if James Bond is your guest) and strain into a cocktail glass. Eschew the tradition of garnishing with an olive, or even a twist of lemon peel, and instead add a slice of cucumber.

LIQUORS

A great way of introducing wild tea flavors into other drinks is to infuse them in liquors. Many of the ingredients in this book will be suitable and the liquors' high alcohol content will quickly get to work extracting the flavors. As a guide, gin lends itself to herbal and floral teas; vodka is a great base for punchy fruit flavors; and some of the spicy chai blends work well in dark rums. Quantities and infusing times will vary greatly according to ingredient, but start with small quantities of liquors and tea, taste test at regular intervals, and have fun experimenting to see what works the best.

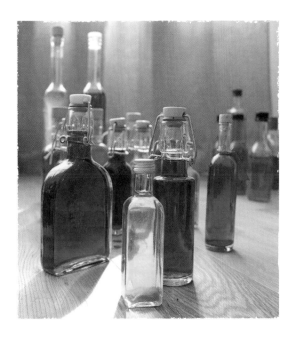

Rich wants to call this a Mar-TEA-ni. Nick isn't so sure.

Strawberry Iced Tea

If you're the kind of person who gets excited by the sight of strawberries, this summertime tea might just set you off on a berry frenzy. It's a quick and easy brew that doesn't require making any syrups—simply pick, blend, chill, and celebrate in the sweet taste of strawberry.

Makes: 4 cups
4 cups water
4 teaspoons black tea or
   4 black tea bags
8 teaspoons sugar (or
   more for a sweet tooth)
Juice of ½ a lemon
1 pound fresh
   strawberries (about
   3 cups chopped), plus
   a few more, to serve

1 Boil 2 cups of water and pour it over the tea and sugar, stirring to dissolve the sugar, and let stand for 5 minutes.

2 Meanwhile, hull and coarsely chop the strawberries, put into a blender, and blend until smooth.

3 When the tea has steeped, strain it into the blended strawberries, stir, and strain them through a fine-mesh strainer. For maximum juice extraction, try pressing the mix with the back of a spoon to force it through the tiny holes.

4 Add the lemon juice and 2 cups of cold water, then refrigerate to chill. Stir before serving, adding ice to your glass and garnishing with a few slices of fresh strawberries.

STRAWBERRY TEA VARIATIONS

Minty Strawberries
Strawberries are one of mint's many admirers. Crush a small handful of fresh leaves (or 2 teaspoons of dried leaves) and add to the tea.

Strawberries and Cream
Strawberries also love vanilla, and for a cream tea without the cream you can add ½ a fresh vanilla bean (or 1 teaspoon of vanilla extract) with the tea bags. If you're desperate for dairy, too, try floating a scoop of ice cream on the top.

Extra Fruity
For an even fruitier ice tea, add some more soft fruit to the strawberries, such as a handful of fresh raspberries.

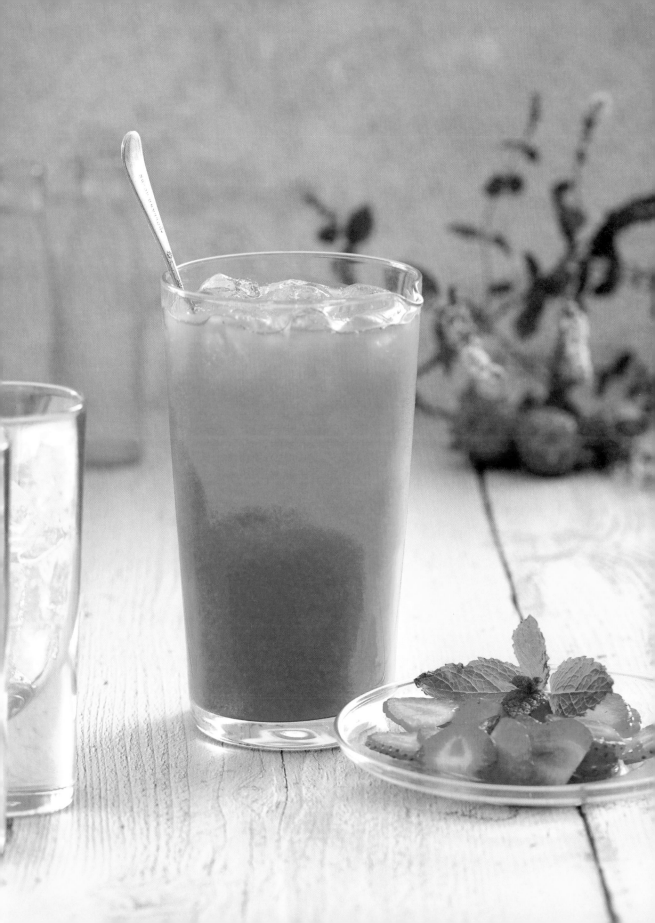

Apple Scraps Tea

We live in an area in England that is famed for its apple growing, and we grow several cultivars ourselves, principally for making cider. This tea is for more sober sipping and is a handy bonus for anyone baking a big apple pie who finds themselves with a mound of leftover apple peels and cores. Apples have varying amounts of tannins in their skins, which gives the tea a refreshing bite, and boiling brings out every last drop of fruity flavor and sugar. It's also a great tea to make with kids who will enjoy transforming curly peels into a tasty drink. Although this recipe works perfectly well with apples alone, it can also be brewed with a flavor partner—we've picked out a few of our favorites for you to try, but why not have some fun and come up with your own ap-peeling combinations?

Makes: 2 cups
Peel and cores from
   5 medium apples
3½ cups water
Brown sugar, honey, or
   maple syrup, to taste

1 Pour the water into a saucepan along with the apple peel and cores and, if you want, one of the optional additions.

2 Bring the pan to a boil and simmer for 10–15 minutes.

3 Strain into a mug and sweeten to taste—sugar or honey are suitable, but we can also recommend a teaspoon of maple syrup.

OPTIONAL ADDITIONS

Spicy apple
Coarsely chop or grate a small thumb-tip-size knob of ginger and add it to the pan.

Fruity apple
Try boiling the mix with about 10 blackberries or raspberries.

Spicy apple
Add ½ a cinnamon stick to the pan with the apple scraps.

Minty apple
Add 5 mint leaves to a mug with the hot liquid.

TOP TIP

Every time you peel an apple, put the scraps into the freezer, ready for when the apple tea mood strikes.

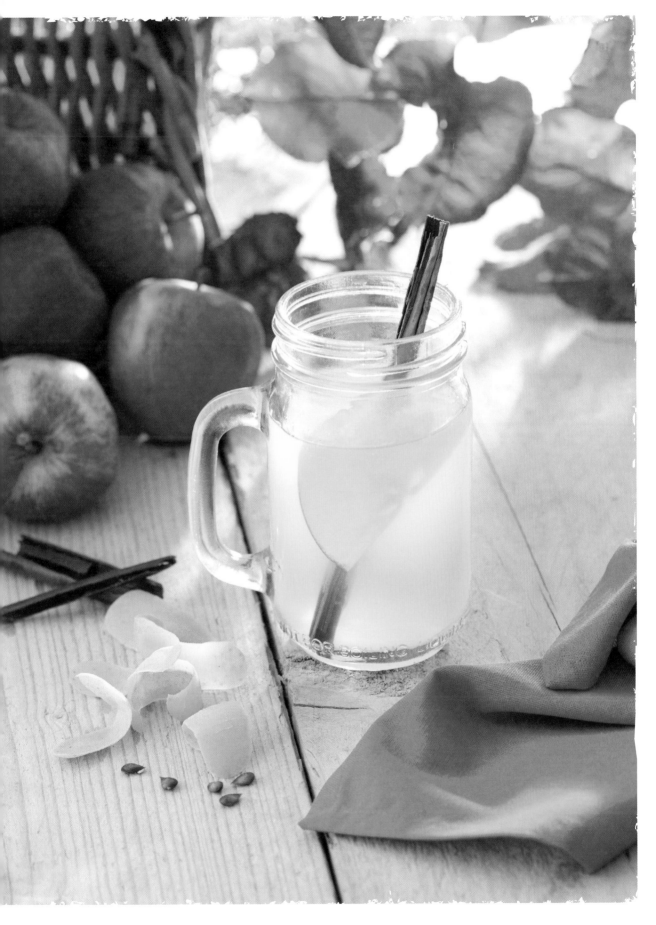

Elderflower and Cucumber Iced Tea

The sight of elderflowers spreading their creamy white blankets of blossom across a sunlit thicket is a sure sign that summer is making its entrance. Those elderflowers make one of the best iced teas around and, in this recipe, we've cooled the temperature down even more by adding cucumber. Clear space in the refrigerator and load up on one of the best tastes of summer.

Makes about 4 cups
12 heads of hand-size
  elderflowers
Juice of 1 lemon
4 cups water
½ cucumber, plus extra,
  to serve
8 teaspoons sugar (or
  more for a sweet
  tooth)
4 teaspoons green tea
  (or 4 green tea bags)

CUCUMBER GARNISHES

For an alternative garnish, try using borage flowers or the young leaves of salad burnet, both of which have a distinctive cucumber-like flavor.

1 First shake your elderflower heads and rinse well to remove any tiny bugs, then separate the flowers into a heatproof bowl— snipping with scissors or rubbing them off between finger and thumb are both suitable methods. A few tiny stalks joining them is fine, but they contain bitter toxins, so you don't want to add too many. Add the lemon juice.

2 Bring 2½ cups of water to a boil, pour it over the elderflowers, cover, and let sit overnight.

3 The next day, peel half a cucumber and coarsely chop into chunks. Put the sugar into a saucepan with 1⅔ cups water and bring to a boil, stirring to dissolve the sugar.

4 When the water reaches boiling point, remove it from the heat and add the cucumber. Let it sit for 2 minutes so that it cools slightly, then add the green tea and let infuse for another 10 minutes.

5 Combine the cucumber and green tea mix with the elderflower mix, then strain into a pitcher (you'll need a fine-mesh strainer or cheesecloth for this task). Refrigerate for at least 1 hour, until chilled.

6 To serve, you can add slices of cucumber and mint leaves as a final flourish of freshness before enjoying the coolest of summer drinks.

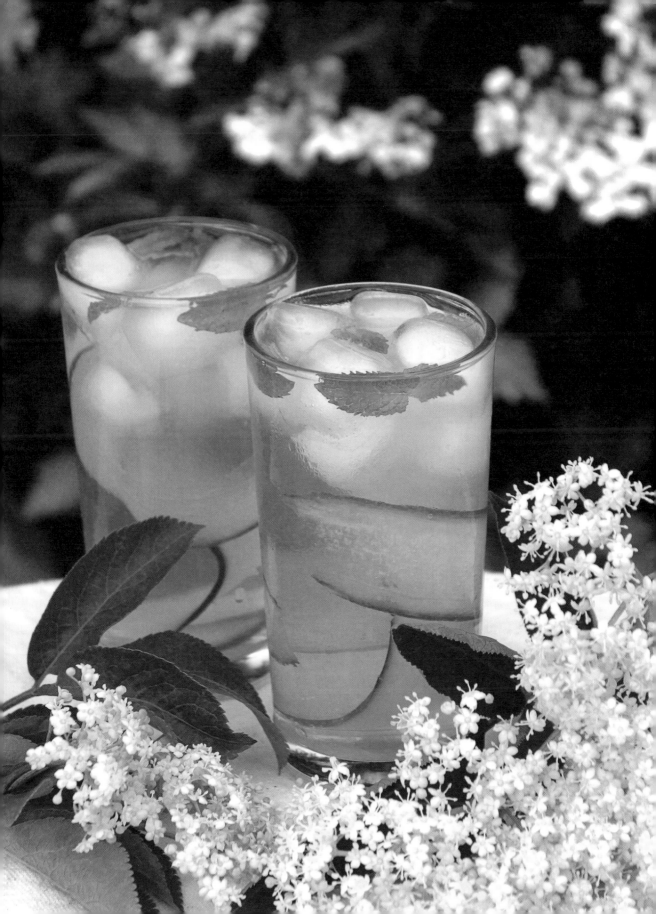

Kombucha

A sweet and sour bubbly tea sounds wrong on many levels, but this probiotic beverage of uncertain Eastern origin can provide a great platform for your wild tea experiments. It's produced by adding a live yeast culture called a scoby* (also referred to as a mother) to a sweet tea mixture. The scoby will snack on the sugary tea, producing a small amount of alcohol and lending the beverage a light sparkle. The following recipe describes how to make a basic black tea kombucha, but you can use whatever tea blend you want, just as long as at least a quarter of the blend is black tea. Leaf through the pages of this book and let your imagination run wild.

Makes: 10 cups
10 cups water
4 teaspoons black tea (or black tea mix)
1 cup sugar
scoby
1½ cups starter tea
Note: You can use tap water, but it really depends on where you live and the quality of the water supply. Water that has been chlorinated may inhibit your scoby growth, so to play it safe, either use bottled water or boil and cool tap water before use.

Equipment
3-quart glass jar
1 cloth for covering the jar
1 funnel or syphon tube for transferring your kombucha to bottles.

SCOBY AND STARTER TEA

To make your first batch of kombucha, you'll need to get hold of a scoby. Either get one from a kombucha-making friend or search online—health food stores may be able to point you in the right direction. A "starter tea" is usually an amount of liquid taken from your previous batch of kombucha, but you can purchase store-bought scobys that are supplied with a premade starter tea.

METHOD

1 Bring 4 cupsof water to a boil, then turn off the heat and add the black tea.

2 Let steep for 5–10 minutes, strain, then add the sugar and stir until dissolved.

3 Add the sugary tea to a 3-quart jar and top off with 5½ cups of cold water—make sure there is at least 2 inches clear at the top for the starter tea and scoby and extra space for fermentation activity. Cover and let cool to room temperature.

4 Add the scoby and starter tea, stir with a wooden spoon, cover the jar with a cloth, and secure with an elastic band. Keep the jar somewhere warm but out of direct sun—a kitchen shelf is ideal.

5 Wait for 7 days, then taste. If your brew tastes too sweet, cover it and continue fermentation so that the sugar content continues to reduce. By 3 weeks, your kombucha should have peaked and will taste tart.

* Or SCOBY—often written in capitals because it is an acronym for Symbiotic Culture Of Bacteria and Yeast. We've kept it lower case, because we didn't want you to think we were shouting.

SCOBY HOTELS

Once introduced to your kombucha, your scoby will expand, grow, and form new scobys. Separate and transfer these to a "scoby hotel"—a jar containing kombucha liquid where your scobys can thrive. Every month or so, you'll want to discard some of the liquid and top it off with sweet tea (see steps 1 and 2). Don't refrigerate it or let your scobys dry out, and discard any scobys that turn black.

6 When the kombucha reaches your desired taste, lift out your scoby and either place it in a scoby hotel (see above) or immediately set it to work on your next batch.

7 Using the funnel or syphon tube, transfer your kombucha to sterilized swing-top bottles, leaving ½–¾ inch of headspace.

8 For further customization, you can add additional flavorings to each bottle. Try adding a fruity syrup, some fresh herbs, or a couple of tablespoons of crushed or chopped fruits, such as strawberries.

9 Keep the bottles at room temperature for 1–3 days. A secondary fermentation will start to occur that will bring added sparkle to your drink. Release any excess CO_2 buildup by opening the caps on your bottles once daily.

10 Store your finished kombucha in the refrigerator. It should keep for 1–2 months.

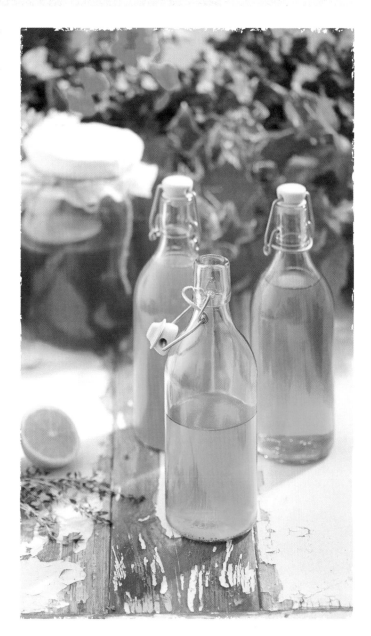

Bubble Tea

You could be forgiven for thinking that this quirky beverage was born of the Instagram generation, but Bubble Tea is no fleeting modern fad. It sprang up in Taiwan in the 1980s and has slowly gained worldwide popularity, thanks to the numerous, customizable flavor combinations it offers, and the addition of boba—either chewy tapioca pearls or bursting spheres of juice or syrup. For the experimental tea maker looking for something a little different, this tea and tapioca tryst provides the ideal canvas for wild creations.

BUBBLE TEA BASICS

Bubble tea can essentially be broken down into three basic styles, with each one offering plenty of opportunities for customization. Follow the rough quantities given right and adjust the milk/tea ratios to your preferred taste. If you prefer a lighter, fresher brew, swap the black tea for green tea.

PLAIN BUBBLE TEA

Makes: 1 cup
1 cup of cold black tea or flavored iced tea
1 lemon slice
3–4 ice cubes

Combine and shake vigorously to blend before filling with the boba of your choice.

MILK BUBBLE TEA

Makes: 1 cup
1 cup of cold black tea
½ cup milk (or milk substitute, see *pages 24–25*)
3–4 ice cubes

Combine and shake vigorously to blend before filling with the boba of your choice.

NOTE

Some of the more acidic fruity additions may curdle your milk, depending on which type you choose. Citrus fruit is especially guilty of this. If curdling occurs, either change the syrup, forgo the milk, or simply suck it up.

FRUITY BUBBLE TEA

Makes: 1 cup
1 cup of cold black tea
Fruity syrup to taste (see *page 166*)
3–4 ice cubes

Combine and shake vigorously to blend before filling with the boba of your choice.

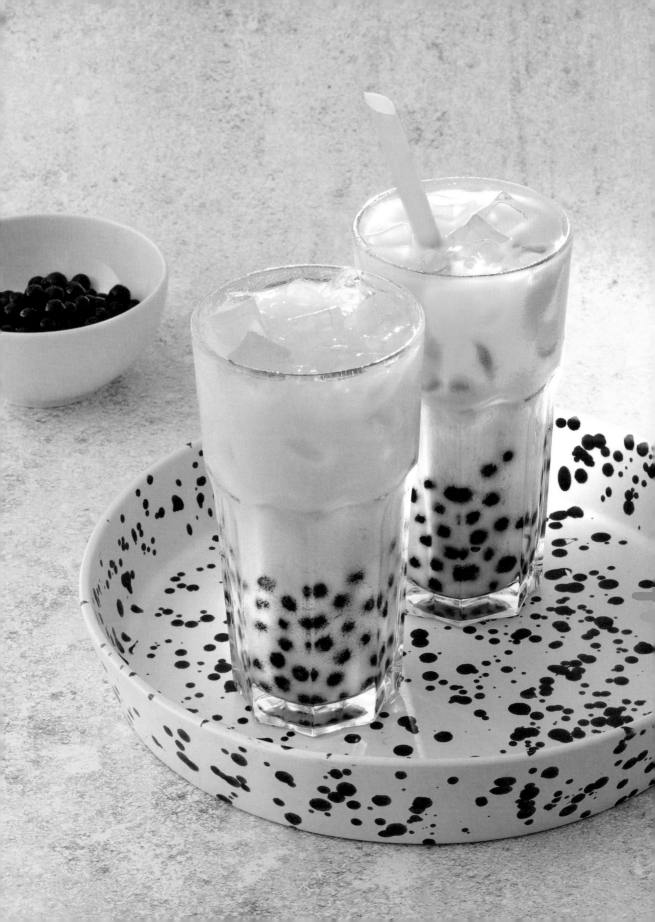

BOBA ADDITIONS FOR BUBBLE TEA

To provide that all-important texture, just add boba. The two most common types are tapioca pearls and the slightly more labor-intensive popping boba. Here's how to make them:

TAPIOCA PEARLS

Although it's possible to make your own tapioca pearls from scratch, we'd recommend purchasing a package of dried ones. Search for them in your local Asian grocery store. Failing that, venture online, where you will find plenty of willing vendors.

Makes: 1 large cup
1 cup of tapioca pearls
10 cups of water
Honey or syrup, for sweetening

To prepare them, add your pearls to a saucepan of boiling water (you'll need 10 cups of water for every cup of pearls) and wait until they rise to the surface. Stir them and continue boiling for 2–3 minutes, then reduce the heat and simmer for another 2–3 minutes. Scoop out the tapioca pearls, plunge them in cold water for 20 seconds, then drain. Mix the pearls with honey or syrup for sweetening and flavor before adding to your cup of bubble tea.

DID YOU KNOW?

Tapioca pearls are made from an extract derived from the roots of the cassava plant, a woody shrub native to South America. The cassava plant must be prepared carefully when processing (which should involve peeling, slicing, then cooking), because raw cassava contains a naturally occurring cyanide.

POPPING BOBA

It's a little more work to make popping boba, but the end results are worth the effort. This "reverse spherification" technique involves encasing your chosen syrup or flavoring with a gelatinous membrane that bursts when bitten into. The ingredients can be found online.

Makes: 1 large cup
4 cups distilled water
2½ teaspoons sodium alginate
½ cup syrup of your choice (see *page 166*)
⅔ teaspoon calcium lactate
Xanthan gum (optional)

1 Grab a mixing bowl and pour in 4 cups of distilled water, then add the sodium alginate.

2 Using a blender, mix for 5–10 minutes, then refrigerate for about 30 minutes to be sure the alginate hydrates properly.

3 In a separate bowl, pour in the syrup and add the calcium lactate (and xantham gum, if using, see step 4). Stir vigorously to combine.

4 Carefully drip blobs of the mixture into the alginate bath, using a spoon or a large syringe from a height just above the surface of the bath. Stir the newly formed spheres carefully with a slotted spoon, then after 30 seconds, transfer them to the rinsing bath.

Your first attempts will probably look like Satan's frogspawn, but with some practice you should be able to make decent spheres. If you keep getting oddly shaped boba, your flavoring mixture may need thickening. Try adding a small amount of xanthan gum in step 3 until the mixture is viscous.

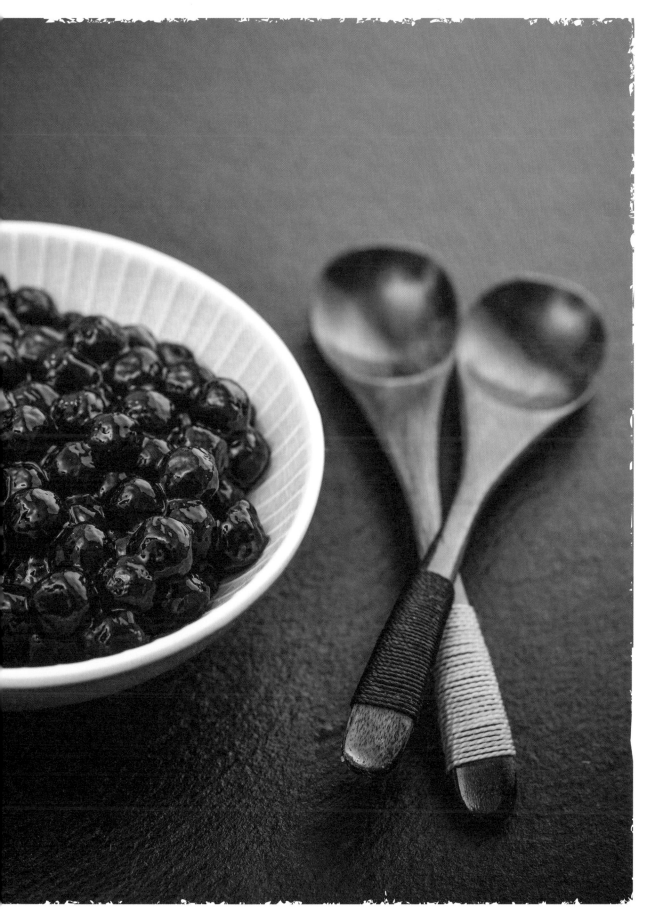

FOUR EASY-TO-MAKE
GARDEN-FORAGED SYRUPS FOR BUBBLE TEA

Here are four fruity syrups to incorporate into your bubble tea experiments. You can also use them to pour over ice cream, and they make great cocktail additions to a gin and tonic or a similarly summery, liquor-based concoction.

WOODRUFF SYRUP

Folk familiar with the insides of German beer halls will probably have seen this syrup accompanying a Berliner Weisse, to which it adds a strawlike sweetness. Green food coloring is often added to woodruff syrup to give it a punchy green hue.

Makes: 1 bottle
1 bunch of sweet woodruff
2½ cups water
1½ cups superfine sugar
2 lemons, washed and sliced
Green food coloring (optional)

1 Wash the woodruff, pat it dry, and let wilt for a day or so to intensify the flavor.

2 Add the water and sugar to a saucepan and bring to a boil. Reduce the heat and simmer to dissolve the sugar, then let cool.

3 Pluck the leaves from the woodruff and add them to the pan. Add the sliced lemons, then cover and chill for a couple of days in the refrigerator.

4 Strain the syrup through a cheesecloth. Return it to a pan and bring to a boil, then remove from the heat. Let cool before pouring into sterilized bottles, adding food coloring, if you want.

ROSE HIP SYRUP

This is without question one of the finest wild syrups you could ever hope to make. Pour it in your tea, pour on pancakes, or just drink it straight like a filthy animal.

Makes: 1 bottle
4 cups rose hips, coarsely chopped
2½ cups water
1½ cups superfine sugar
Juice of 1 lemon

1 Mash up your rose hips using a mortar and pestle or similar, then put into a saucepan with the water. Bring to a boil, then simmer for 15 minutes.

2 Remove from the heat, then strain through a cheesecloth into another saucepan, squeezing it if necessary.

3 Strain again through a clean cheesecloth to be sure no irritating rose hip hairs make their way into the final syrup.

4 Add the sugar, then bring to a boil, stirring until the sugar has dissolved. Continue to boil for another 5 minutes, skimming off any scum that rises with a spoon.

5 Pour into sterilized bottles when cool.

TOP TIP

When refrigerated, your syrups should last for a month or so. Shake them before use if the liquid has started to separate. Adding 1 teaspoon of vodka when bottling will extend their shelf life to about 6 months.

RHUBARB AND GINGER SYRUP

Don't just save it for a tart or pie—turn your rhubarb stash into a pink-hued syrup for your bubble tea experiments. Mix with tapioca pearls and a slice of vanilla bean for a bubble tea take on rhubarb and custard.

Makes: 1 bottle
1 pound rhubarb stalks
2½ cups water
Juice of 1 lemon
1½ cups superfine sugar
1 knob of fresh ginger, grated

1 Chop the rhubarb into 1-inch chunks and put into a large saucepan with the water, lemon juice, sugar, and ginger.

2 Bring to a boil and simmer for about 30 minutes, until the rhubarb turns pulpy.

3 Remove from the heat and strain through a cheesecloth into another saucepan or suitable container. You might need to squeeze the bag a little to encourage the juices to flow, but beware that the bag and contents will be HOT. Suspend the bag and let it drip for a few hours, if possible.

4 Pour into sterilized bottles when cool.

LEMON BALM SYRUP

This tart, lemon-flavored syrup is perfect for summertime slurping. You can try this one with a bubble tea base made from chamomile instead of black tea.

Makes: 1 bottle
2½ cups water
1½ cups superfine sugar
1 large handful of lemon balm leaves
Juice of 1 lemon

1 Add the water and sugar to a saucepan and bring to a boil, stirring until the sugar has dissolved. Reduce the heat to a simmer.

2 Add the lemon balm leaves and lemon juice and continue to simmer for about 10 minutes.

3 Strain through a cheesecloth and pour into sterilized bottles when cool.

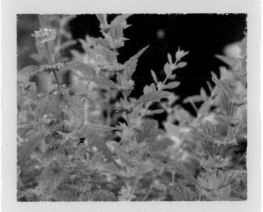

Wild Coffee

For a wild alternative to the country's favorite pick-me-up, head outdoors with your finest foraging bag and get gathering. The nuts, roots, and seeds on this page offer surprisingly tasty "real" coffee alternatives, packed with slightly bitter, roasted flavors, and they provide instant success without the alarming price tag. The only real difference is the lack of caffeine—which can be a bonus or a curse, depending on which way you look at it.

DANDELION COFFEE

Who would have thought that the roots of this tenacious lawn-loving plant could produce such a tasty brew? You shouldn't have much trouble sourcing willing plants—a quick trip to our unkempt garden will often yield enough to make a tray-load of steaming beverages.

Serve: 1–2 teaspoons per cup

1 Dig up your dandelion roots, scrub, and let dry on a warm windowsill.

2 Break or chop up your roots into small pieces.

3 Roast on a baking sheet in a preheated oven at 400°F for 30–40 minutes, until brittle, then grind them up with a pestle and mortar, if you have one (a rolling pin/bowl combo will work just as well).

4 Use 1–2 teaspoons per cup of boiling water. Let infuse for 5 minutes before straining and serving.

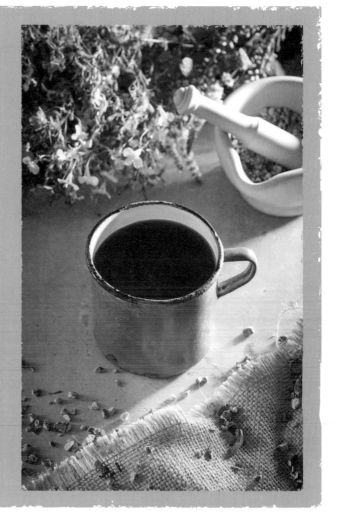

CLEAVERS COFFEE

Cleavers (also known as goosegrass or sticky willy) make a fine coffee substitute. We'd argue that it tastes even better than dandelion coffee, albeit much more hassle to harvest. You'll need to gather a lot—the plant-to-seed ratio is stacked considerably against the latter and it's the hairy seeds that you need. The resulting brew smells just like a freshly ground coffee; the taste is a kind of black tea/coffee crossover.

Serve: 1–2 teaspoons per cup

1 The best way to gather cleavers is to grab handfuls of the plant—stem and all—and let dry out overnight. The seeds will then detach more easily from the stems.

2 Spread a thin layer of seeds on a baking sheet and roast for 20 minutes at 400°F.

3 Grind them up the best you can with a mortar and pestle.

4 Use 1–2 teaspoons per cup of boiling water. Let infuse for 5 minutes, then strain and serve.

ACORN COFFEE

Acorn coffee was used as a substitute during World War II when supplies of the real thing were scarce, and rumor has it that unscrupulous coffee makers would cut their stocks with this nutty alternative to boost profits. Compared to dandelion coffee, acorn coffee takes more effort to make, because acorns are bitter and therefore first need boiling to tame the tannins. It's still worth trying, however, if you happen to have a lot of nuts.

Serve: 1–2 teaspoons per cup

1 Add the acorns to a saucepan, cover with water, and bring to a boil, then simmer for 15–20 minutes.

2 Let cool, then remove the hard outer shells with a sharp knife, being careful to avoid slicing your fingers.

3 Roast on a baking sheet in a preheated oven at 400°F for 30–40 minutes, until brown and fragrant.

4 Chop the roasted nuts in a food processor, then return to the oven for 20 minutes.

5 Give them a final grind with a mortar and pestle.

6 Use 1–2 teaspoons per cup of boiling water. Let infuse for 5 minutes before straining and serving.

CHICORY COFFEE

Not to be confused with the leafy bitter vegetable of the same name, this coffee impostor is made from the roots of the blue-flowered herb *Cichorium intybus*—a close relative of the dandelion. Camp Coffee, the bottled coffee-flavored syrup, is made using chicory and became popular during the 1970s when real coffee prices soared due to crop-spoiling frosts in Brazil.

Serve: 1–2 teaspoons per cup

1 Pull up your chicory, separate the roots from the plant, scrub, and set aside to dry.

2 Break or chop up your roots into small pieces.

3 Roast on a baking sheet in a preheated oven at 400°F for 30–40 minutes, until brittle, then grind well using a mortar and pestle.

4 Use 1–2 teaspoons per cup of boiling water. Let infuse for 5 minutes before straining and serving.

Hazelnut Latte

We both studied at Coventry School of Art and Design in the early 1990s—
innocent days before Starbucks had crashed the scene, and when coffee
served in the city center precinct came in two types: with or without milk.
Asking for a hazelnut latte back then would have resulted in quizzical looks
and laughter, but nowadays you'll often hear its name barked at baristas
in hipster coffee shops. Hazelnut syrup (the crucial ingredient) is readily
available in most grocery stores, but we think our homemade recipe will
knock your socks off. For that authentic coffee shop vibe, drink it from
a paper cup with your name spelled incorrectly down the side.

Syrup
1 cup hazelnuts,
   blanched and roasted
   (see box)
1 cup water
2 tablespoons honey
⅔ cup tightly packed
   light brown sugar

Latte
Makes: 1 large mug
strong black coffee and
   milk (dairy or non-dairy,
   see *pages 24–25*)

TO MAKE THE SYRUP

1 Wrap the hazelnuts in a clean
kitchen towel or plastic bag and
pummel them into small pieces
using a rolling pin or suitably
heavy implement.

2 Pour the water into a saucepan,
bring to a boil, then stir in the
honey and brown sugar until
dissolved.

3 Add the smashed nuts, reduce the
heat, and simmer for 15 minutes.
Stir occasionally so they don't burn
on the bottom of the pan.

4 Strain the resulting mixture
through a cheesecloth or strainer
into sterilized bottles. It's good
practice to let liquids cool before
pouring into glass bottles or they
may crack. Plus there's a good
chance you'll scald your hands on
the lava-hot liquid. Store your
filled bottles in the refrigerator.

5 Don't throw out the leftover
nuts—you can use them to top
your morning bowl of porridge for
a nutty bonus.

TO MAKE THE HAZELNUT LATTE

1 Fill a mug halway with a strong
black coffee of your choice (see
pages 168–169 for some foraged
alternatives).

2 Top off with warm milk.

3 Add 2–3 teaspoons hazelnut
syrup (or to taste) and enjoy!

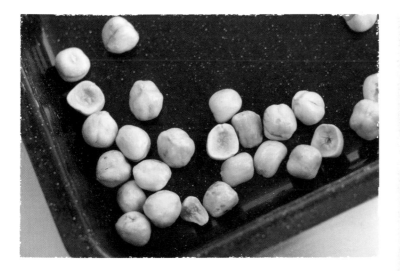

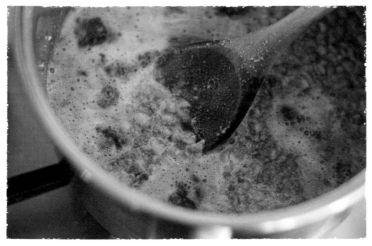

HOW TO BLANCH AND ROAST HAZELNUTS

2 cups water
1 cup hazelnuts
2 tablespoons baking soda

To rid your hazelnuts of their bitter, papery skins you'll need to blanch them as below.

1 Preheat the oven to 350°F.

2 Bring 2 cups of water to a boil in a saucepan, plunge in your hazelnuts, and add the baking soda. Boil on the stove for 4–5 minutes.

3 Remove from the heat, strain the nuts in a colander, and rinse thoroughly in cold water. They'll look like a big pile of rotten molars, but don't worry.

4 Remove the skins from the nuts by rubbing them with your fingers. When they've come off, rinse again under cold water and dry them with a dish towel or similar.

5 Put your skinless hazelnuts onto a baking sheet and roast them in the oven for about 15 minutes, until golden brown.

6 Stand back and admire your lovely nuts. Store them in an airtight container for up to 6 months.

HARVESTING HAZELNUTS

Hazelnuts (also known as cobnuts) should be ready to harvest in late summer or early fall. Although they are best picked when ripe, you'll often find that squirrels will have gotten there before you have a chance to fill your foraging bag. Beat them to it by picking the nuts while still green and storing them to ripen. Keep them inside a cardboard box somewhere dark, warm, and dry. Store them for a couple of weeks, shaking the box occasionally, and wait until the nuts separate readily from their cases. Remember to remove the outer shell before use.

Blackberry Frappé

Here's our wild take on a Greek frappé, the frozen frothy coffee designed for summertime sipping. It's a beverage that requires some vigorous mixing—we use a cocktail shaker for style and swagger, but novice baristas may want to err on the side of caution. A shaker packed with frappé can lead to unexpected kitchen spillages, so to prevent a Greek tragedy, pay attention to the box on the facing page.

Syrup
3½ cups blackberries
1⅔ cups water
1 cup superfine sugar

Frappé
Makes: 1 large mug
1 cup strong black coffee
   or coffee substitute
   (see *pages 168–169*),
   chilled
½ cup milk of choice
   (see *pages 24–25*)
4–5 ice cubes
1 generous scoop of soft
   vanilla ice cream
3 tablespoons
   blackberry syrup
Whipped cream, to serve

TO MAKE THE SYRUP

1 Put your blackberries into a saucepan, add water, and bring to a boil.

2 Put a lid onto the pan and simmer for 30 minutes, or until the fruit turns into mush. To help the process, mash them with a potato masher.

3 Remove from the heat, then strain through a cheesecloth into a saucepan. It may take a while for the pulpy mix to give up its juice, so suspend the bag and let it drip, if you can.

4 When all of the juice is in the pan, add the sugar, stir it, and bring to a boil.

5 Stir until the sugar is dissolved. Continue to simmer for 5 minutes, then set aside to cool. Pour into sterilized bottles; it will keep for about 1 month in the refrigerator.

TO MAKE THE BLACKBERRY FRAPPÉ

1 Pour the coffee into a cocktail shaker and add the milk, ice cubes, and ice cream. Add the syrup (use more or less, depending on taste).

2 Shake it vigorously for about 30 seconds, until the ice is smashed and the milky coffee is foamy.

3 Pour into a large glass and add a straw. Top with a dollop of whipped cream, if you want.

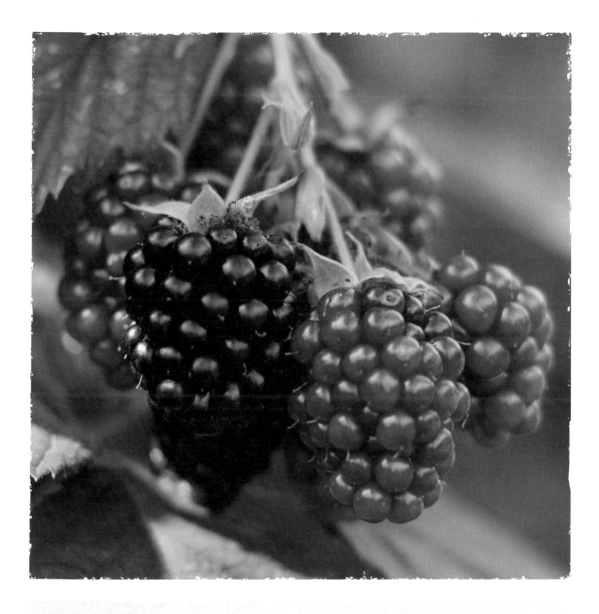

OUR TOP TIPS ON COCKTAIL SHAKING

1. Shake It Firmly

Hold your shaker with both hands, one supporting the bottom and one gripping the neck, with fingers curled firmly over the lid.

2. Shake It Hard, Shake It Long

Don't be shy, shake it well. Expect to shake for about 20 seconds. If you are using a smart stainless steel shaker, the outside will form frost, letting you know the contents are ready for pouring.

3. Shake It Safe

If you have been ignoring step 1 and the lid of the shaker flies off, shaking over your shoulder will ensure that your guests aren't showered in frappé. Speaking from experience, blackberry frappé doesn't wash out of clothes all that well.

Index

Acknowledgments

Big thanks to everyone who helped us make this book happen, in particular Dave Hamilton for his expert foraging advice and Jane Moore at The Bath Priory for her growing know-how and the photo opportunities her immaculate garden provided. We would also like to thank our foreign correspondents Nagahiro Yasumori, Natsuki Kikuya and Wendy Dewar, as well as those who supplied invaluable knowledge closer to home— Sue Mullet of Bath Botanicals, Meghan and Rob at St Austell Brewery and the good folk of St Ives Gin.

Thanks to our agent Jane for connecting us with Lisa Dyer at Eddison Books, who has been full of advice and encouragement, and everyone else involved in the production of the book, including Nicolette Kaponis, Grace Paul, Anna Cheifetz, Ruth Jenkinson (photography) and James Pople (design). Other people we would like to mention for their assistance and support are Becky, Liz and Lenny, Emman Depau and Lyndsey Mayhew.

Finally, Rich would especially like to thank Catherine, Daisy, Emily and Annabel and Nick has oodles of extra gratitude for Kerry and Flynn—all for helping us to pick, brew and taste. We promise to never again ask you to try mallow tea (although we can't promise there will be no more stinky seaweed experiments).

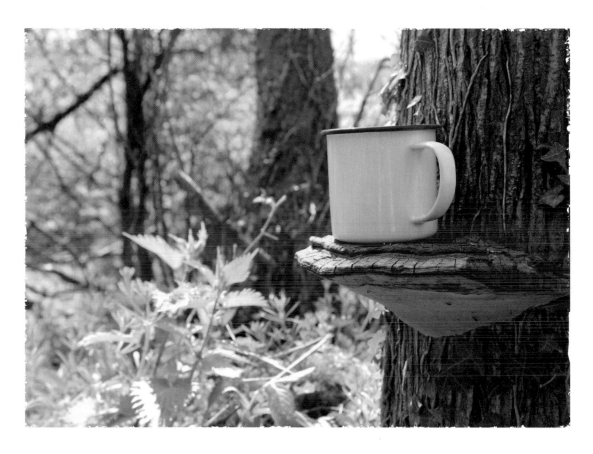